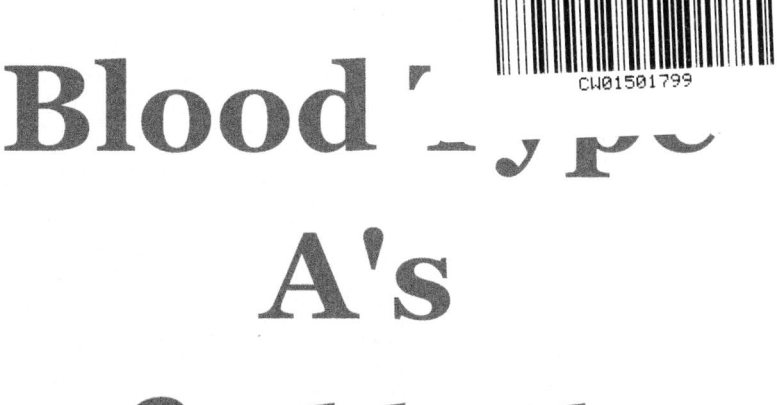

Blood Type

A's

Cookbook

A Blood Type Diet Book for A-Positive and Negative - Customized Delicious and Nutritious Recipes and Insights for Healthy Living.

Georgina hayes

Dedication

This cookbook is dedicated to all the health-conscious individuals with Blood Type A-Positive and A-Negative, who are committed to nourishing their bodies and embracing a healthier lifestyle. May this collection of nutritious and delectable recipes bring joy, inspiration, and fulfillment to your culinary journey. Here's to a life filled with vibrant health, delicious meals, and the joy of cooking!

Table of contents

Part 1:
A-Positive

Introduction

Welcome to the captivating world of "Blood Type A's Cookbook: Customized Delicious and Nutritious Recipes and Insights for Healthy Living." Here, we embark on a journey that celebrates the harmonious relationship between food and well-being, tailored exclusively for A-Positive and A-Negative individuals.

Have you ever wondered why certain diets work wonders for some people, while others find them less effective? The answer may lie in our unique blood types—a defining aspect of our biology that influences how our bodies respond to different foods. Blood Type A, in particular, boasts a distinct set of traits that can be nourished and supported through a personalized dietary approach.

In this cookbook, we dive deep into the realm of the Blood Type Diet, focusing on individuals with A-Positive and A-Negative blood types. As we explore the landscape of nutrition, you'll come to appreciate the significance of customizing your diet to your blood type, unlocking a world of benefits for your overall health.

A Glimpse into the Journey Ahead:

At the heart of this culinary expedition, you'll find an array of tantalizing recipes meticulously crafted to resonate harmoniously with the unique needs of Blood Type A individuals. From the invigorating breakfasts that greet your mornings to the comforting dinners that bid you goodnight, each recipe is an invitation to embrace the goodness of wholesome, flavorful ingredients.

But it's not just about the delicious fare. The magic lies in the tailored nutrition that supports your body's innate tendencies. The health benefits associated with aligning your diet with your blood type are truly astounding, transcending mere physical well-being to encompass a profound sense of vitality and balance.

As you turn the pages, you'll find illuminating insights and explanations that deepen your understanding of the Blood Type Diet. We'll walk hand in hand, demystifying the reasons behind specific food choices, and empowering you to make informed decisions about your nutrition.

A Personalized Approach to Wellness:

The beauty of the Blood Type Diet lies in its personalized nature. It acknowledges that we are each uniquely wired, and what suits one may not fit another. By honoring this individuality, we step onto a path of enhanced well-being, one that embraces not just our physical health but also our emotional and mental vitality.

With a spotlight on plant-based goodness, our cookbook revels in the splendor of nature's bounty. Fruits, vegetables, grains, and plant proteins take center stage, showcasing the diversity of flavors and nutrients that await your palate.

A Call to Action: Embrace the Journey

Are you ready to embark on this transformative journey of nourishment and self-discovery? Are you prepared to savor the delights of wholesome cooking tailored to your blood type? If your heart sings a resounding "yes," then take the leap.

With "Blood Type A's Cookbook," you hold the key to unlocking the full potential of your unique biology. The door to a healthier and happier you awaits—step inside and embark on a culinary adventure that celebrates the art of nourishment and the joy of savoring each delectable bite. Your path to vitality and balance begins now.

- Understanding the Blood Type Diet for A-Positive

Before we immerse ourselves in the delightful recipes tailored for A-Positive individuals, let's take a moment to understand the essence of the

Blood Type Diet and how it aligns with your specific blood type.

The Blood Type Diet: A Brief Overview

The concept of the Blood Type Diet was introduced by Dr. Peter J. D'Adamo, a naturopathic physician and author, who proposed that our blood types hold valuable clues to optimal health and nutrition. According to this theory, each blood type (A, B, AB, and O) has unique dietary needs based on the genetic markers inherited from our ancestors.

For individuals with A-Positive blood type, the diet primarily revolves around embracing a more plant-based approach. This means emphasizing a rich array of fruits, vegetables, grains, and legumes, while minimizing or avoiding certain foods that may be less compatible with your biology.

The A-Positive Diet: Key Characteristics

1. **Plant-Based Emphasis:** A-Positive individuals tend to flourish on diets that are

predominantly plant-based. Fresh fruits and vegetables are central to this approach, providing essential vitamins, minerals, and antioxidants to support your well-being.

2. Grains and Legumes: Whole grains, such as quinoa, brown rice, and oats, are excellent staples for A-Positive individuals. Additionally, legumes like lentils, chickpeas, and beans offer valuable plant-based protein sources.

3. Lean Proteins: While plant-based proteins form the foundation of the A-Positive diet, lean animal proteins like poultry and fish can also be included in moderation. Red meat, however, is best limited.

4. Dairy and Beyond: For A-Positive individuals, dairy products are generally best kept in moderation. Opt for alternatives like almond milk, coconut milk, or soy milk if you prefer non-dairy options.

5. Mindful Fats: Healthy fats are essential for overall health, but it's essential to choose wisely. Incorporate sources like avocados, nuts, seeds, and olive oil while reducing or avoiding saturated and trans fats.

The Benefits of Eating for Your Blood Type

You might wonder, "What sets the Blood Type Diet apart from other dietary approaches?" The answer lies in its focus on individualized nutrition. By tailoring your diet to your specific blood type, you may experience a range of benefits, including:

- **Improved Digestion:** When you consume foods that align with your blood type, your digestive system tends to function more efficiently, leading to reduced bloating and discomfort.

- **Enhanced Energy Levels:** A-Positive individuals often report increased energy and vitality when they adopt a diet suited to their blood type, supporting their daily activities with a spring in their step.

- Weight Management: Embracing a diet aligned with your blood type may facilitate weight management by optimizing nutrient absorption and supporting your body's natural metabolic processes.

- Better Immune Function: Nourishing your body with foods that complement your blood type can strengthen your immune system and help you resist common ailments.

Embrace the Journey to a Healthier You

Now that we've unraveled the foundation of the Blood Type Diet for A-Positive individuals, you're primed to explore the enchanting world of culinary creations that await you. Let the adventure begin as we indulge in a delightful assortment of recipes designed to nourish your body and tantalize your taste buds. Embrace the personalized path to wellness and savor the joy of eating in harmony with your unique biology.

- Health Benefits and Considerations for Blood Type A-Positive

As an A-Positive individual, you hold a unique genetic makeup that responds remarkably to a diet tailored to your blood type. Let's delve into the health benefits and considerations of following the Blood Type A Diet, allowing you to thrive and flourish in your journey towards better well-being.

Health Benefits of the Blood Type A Diet:

1. Optimized Digestion: The Blood Type A Diet encourages foods that are easily digestible for A-Positive individuals, reducing the likelihood of digestive discomfort such as bloating, gas, and indigestion.

2. Enhanced Immune Function: By consuming a diet rich in fruits, vegetables, and plant-based proteins, A-Positive individuals can bolster their immune system, helping the body ward off infections and illnesses more effectively.

3. Weight Management: The Blood Type A Diet's emphasis on a plant-based approach, combined with lean proteins, can support healthy weight management for A-Positive individuals.

4. Increased Energy Levels: Eating in harmony with your blood type can lead to a sustained and stable energy level throughout the day, reducing energy fluctuations and fatigue.

5. Heart Health: By avoiding or minimizing red meat and unhealthy fats, A-Positive individuals may experience improved cardiovascular health and reduced risk of heart-related issues.

Considerations for A-Positive Individuals:

1. Moderate Dairy Intake: While some dairy products may be consumed in moderation, A-Positive individuals often benefit from choosing non-dairy alternatives like almond or soy milk.

2. Mindful Protein Choices: Lean poultry and fish are suitable protein options for A-Positive individuals, while red meat and processed meats are best limited due to potential inflammatory effects.

3. Whole Grains and Legumes: Including whole grains and legumes in the diet can provide A-Positive individuals with essential nutrients and plant-based protein sources.

4. Stress Management: A-Positive individuals may be particularly sensitive to stress, so incorporating stress-reduction techniques like meditation, yoga, or mindfulness can support overall well-being.

5. Individual Variations: While the Blood Type A Diet provides general guidelines, it's essential to listen to your body and make adjustments based on your individual needs and preferences.

Embrace the Journey to Optimal Health:

As you embark on this nutritional journey tailored for A-Positive individuals, remember that it's a process of discovery and learning. Embrace the joy of exploring new flavors, experimenting with nourishing ingredients, and savoring each wholesome meal. By aligning your diet with your blood type, you're taking a proactive step towards improved health and well-being—a journey filled with vitality and fulfillment. Let the transformative power of the Blood Type A Diet guide you to a healthier and happier you.

Chapter 1:

The Basics of Blood Type A-Positive Diet

- What Makes Blood Type A-Positive Unique?

Blood Type A-Positive is characterized by the presence of the A antigen and the Rh factor (D antigen) on the surface of red blood cells. This unique combination of genetic markers sets A-Positive individuals apart and influences their physiological and behavioral traits. Here are some key aspects that make A-Positive blood type distinctive:

1. Genetic Expression: A-Positive blood type is the result of specific genetic expressions inherited from ancestors. Historically, this blood type is believed to have emerged in early agricultural societies, adapting to dietary changes related to settled agricultural practices.

2. Personality Traits: A-Positive individuals are often described as empathetic, sensitive, and adaptable. They possess a natural inclination towards understanding the emotions and needs of others and are skilled at navigating complex social situations with grace.

3. Dietary Considerations: The Blood Type A-Positive Diet is designed to align with the unique biological characteristics of A-Positive individuals. It emphasizes a plant-based approach, with a focus on fruits, vegetables, grains, and legumes. Lean proteins, such as poultry and fish, are preferred over red meat.

4. Stress Sensitivity: A-Positive individuals may exhibit increased sensitivity to stress. As such, they may benefit from incorporating stress-reduction techniques and mindfulness practices into their lifestyle.

5. Wellness Focus: A-Positive individuals tend to prioritize their health and well-being. They often seek holistic approaches to maintain physical and emotional balance, embracing a lifestyle that supports their overall wellness.

Understanding what makes A-Positive blood type unique helps individuals make informed choices about their health and nutrition. The Blood Type A-Positive Diet capitalizes on these distinctive traits to create a personalized approach to well-being, optimizing health outcomes and promoting a harmonious and balanced lifestyle. By embracing the tailored recommendations of the Blood Type A-Positive Diet, individuals can embark on a journey of improved vitality and enhanced overall wellness.

- Foods to Emphasize for A-Positive Individuals

The Blood Type A-Positive Diet focuses on providing A-Positive individuals with a nourishing and balanced selection of foods that complement their unique genetic makeup. Here are the key food groups to emphasize in the diet:

1. Abundant Fruits and Vegetables: A-Positive individuals should rejoice in the vibrant world of fruits and vegetables. These nutrient-rich foods provide essential vitamins, minerals, and antioxidants that support overall health. Opt for a colorful variety, including leafy greens, berries, citrus fruits, and cruciferous vegetables like broccoli and cauliflower.

2. Wholesome Grains: Whole grains are a cornerstone of the A-Positive diet. Incorporate nutrient-dense grains such as quinoa, brown rice, oats, and amaranth into your meals. These grains offer sustained energy and support digestive health.

3. Plant Proteins: As A-Positive individuals thrive on plant-based diets, plant proteins take center stage. Enjoy a variety of legumes like lentils, chickpeas, black beans, and edamame. Nuts and seeds also contribute to the protein intake and provide healthy fats.

4. Lean Poultry and Fish: While A-Positive individuals primarily focus on plant-based proteins, lean poultry and fish can be included in moderation. Opt for organic, free-range, or wild-caught options for the best nutritional value.

5. Healthy Fats: Incorporate heart-healthy fats into your diet through sources like avocados, olive oil, flaxseed, and chia seeds. These fats support brain health, skin elasticity, and overall well-being.

6. Dairy Alternatives: A-Positive individuals may choose dairy alternatives like almond milk, coconut milk, or soy milk. If you prefer dairy, opt for low-fat or organic options in moderation.

7. Herbs and Spices: Flavor your meals with a variety of herbs and spices. These not only enhance taste but also provide additional health benefits. Include turmeric, ginger, garlic, basil, and oregano in your culinary creations.

8. Natural Sweeteners: When indulging your sweet tooth, opt for natural sweeteners like honey, maple syrup, or stevia. These alternatives provide a touch of sweetness without causing sharp spikes in blood sugar levels.

Remember, the key to the A-Positive diet is variety and balance. Experiment with different combinations of fruits, vegetables, grains, and proteins to create an enticing array of flavors on your plate. Emphasizing these wholesome foods aligns with your unique biology and can promote optimal health and well-being for A-Positive individuals. Enjoy the journey of nourishing yourself with delicious, healthful meals that celebrate the art of eating for your blood type.

- Foods to Avoid or Limit for A-Positive Individuals

In the Blood Type A-Positive Diet, certain foods may be less compatible with the unique biology of A-Positive individuals. Here are the foods that are best avoided or limited:

1. Red Meat: A-Positive individuals are advised to limit their consumption of red meat, including beef, pork, and lamb. These meats may lead to increased levels of cortisol, the stress hormone, and potentially contribute to inflammation.

2. Processed Meats: Processed meats like bacon, sausage, and deli meats should be avoided or minimized. These foods are often high in preservatives, sodium, and unhealthy fats, which can be detrimental to overall health.

3. High-Fat Dairy: Full-fat dairy products may not be well-tolerated by some A-Positive individuals. Limit consumption of whole milk, full-fat cheese, and butter. Instead, opt for low-fat or non-dairy alternatives.

4. Certain Grains: While many grains are beneficial, some may not be as well-suited for A-Positive individuals. Limit your intake of wheat and products containing wheat, as well as refined grains like white rice and white bread.

5. Corn and Tomatoes: For some A-Positive individuals, corn and tomatoes may cause adverse reactions. Pay attention to how your body responds to these foods and consider reducing or eliminating them if necessary.

6. Highly Processed Foods: Processed foods, such as packaged snacks, sugary treats, and fast food, should be avoided. These foods are often loaded with artificial additives, preservatives, and unhealthy fats.

7. Certain Legumes: While most legumes are encouraged in the A-Positive Diet, some individuals may experience difficulty digesting specific types, such as kidney beans or black-eyed peas. Observe your body's response and adjust accordingly.

8. Sugary Beverages: Sugary sodas, fruit juices with added sugars, and sweetened beverages should be limited or avoided. Opt for water, herbal teas, or naturally flavored water to stay hydrated.

9. Caffeine and Alcohol: Caffeinated beverages and alcohol may have varying effects on A-Positive individuals. Some may tolerate them in moderation, while others may prefer to limit or avoid them altogether.

10. Nightshade Vegetables: Nightshade vegetables, such as eggplants, peppers, and potatoes, may cause sensitivity in some A-Positive individuals. Pay attention to how your body reacts to these foods.

Personalization is Key:

It's essential to remember that the Blood Type A-Positive Diet provides general guidelines, but each individual's response to specific foods can vary. Pay attention to how your body feels after consuming certain foods and make adjustments accordingly. By tailoring your diet to suit your unique needs, you can optimize your health and well-being on your journey to a balanced and nourished lifestyle.

Chapter 2:

Breakfast Delights

- Superfood Smoothie Bowl

Start your day on a vibrant and nourishing note with this delightful Superfood Smoothie Bowl. Packed with essential nutrients and energizing flavors, this breakfast treat will leave you feeling refreshed and ready to take on the day ahead. Let's walk through the steps to create this scrumptious and healthful bowl of goodness:

Ingredients:
- 1 ripe banana, frozen
- 1/2 cup mixed berries (such as blueberries, strawberries, or raspberries), frozen
- 1/2 cup spinach or kale leaves, fresh or frozen
- 1 tablespoon chia seeds
- 1 tablespoon almond butter or peanut butter
- 1/2 cup unsweetened almond milk or coconut milk

- Toppings of your choice (e.g., sliced fruits, granola, coconut flakes, nuts, seeds)

Health Tip: The Healthy Components of the Major Ingredients

Let's take a closer look at the major ingredients in this Superfood Smoothie Bowl and discover the health benefits they bring to your breakfast:

1. Banana: Rich in potassium, fiber, and essential vitamins, bananas are a powerhouse of nutrients. Potassium helps regulate blood pressure, while the fiber aids in digestion and promotes a feeling of fullness, making it a satisfying and heart-healthy addition to your smoothie bowl.

2. Mixed Berries: Bursting with antioxidants, vitamins, and fiber, mixed berries add a burst of color and flavor to your smoothie bowl. Berries like blueberries, strawberries, and raspberries offer a range of health benefits, including immune support, improved heart health, and enhanced cognitive function.

3. Spinach or Kale: Leafy greens like spinach or kale are nutritional powerhouses, providing an abundance of vitamins A, C, K, and minerals like iron and calcium. Incorporating greens into your smoothie bowl boosts your daily nutrient intake and supports overall vitality.

4. Chia Seeds: These tiny seeds are rich in omega-3 fatty acids, fiber, and protein. They help promote a feeling of fullness and aid in digestion. Chia seeds also contribute to stable energy levels, making them a valuable addition to your morning meal.

5. Almond Butter or Peanut Butter: Nut butters offer healthy fats, protein, and a range of essential nutrients. Whether you choose almond butter or peanut butter, you'll benefit from their heart-healthy monounsaturated fats, supporting brain function and satiety.

6. Unsweetened Almond Milk or Coconut Milk: Using unsweetened almond milk or coconut milk keeps your smoothie bowl light and dairy-free. Both options provide calcium, vitamin D, and vitamin E, contributing to strong bones and skin health.

Instructions:

Step 1: Gather all the ingredients and ensure the banana and mixed berries are frozen. Freezing the fruits not only adds a refreshing chill to the smoothie but also gives it a creamy consistency.

Step 2: In a high-speed blender, add the frozen banana, mixed berries, spinach or kale leaves, chia seeds, almond butter or peanut butter, and unsweetened almond milk or coconut milk.

Step 3: Blend until you achieve a smooth and creamy texture. You may need to stop and scrape down the sides of the blender to ensure all the ingredients are well incorporated.

Step 4: Pour the smoothie into a bowl and get creative with your toppings! Sliced fruits, crunchy granola, coconut flakes, nuts, and seeds add texture and additional nutrients to your bowl.

Step 5: Sit back, take in the beautiful colors and textures of your Superfood Smoothie Bowl, and savor each spoonful mindfully. Enjoy the nourishment and energy this nutritious breakfast provides, setting the tone for a vibrant and fulfilling day ahead.

- Veggie-Packed Frittata

Kickstart your morning with a delicious and nutrient-rich Veggie-Packed Frittata. This savory egg dish is a perfect way to incorporate an assortment of colorful vegetables into your breakfast, providing you with a hearty and satisfying meal to fuel your day. Let's dive into the recipe and discover the wholesome goodness of this frittata:

Ingredients:
- 6 large eggs
- 1/4 cup milk (dairy or plant-based)
- 1 cup diced bell peppers (assorted colors)
- 1 cup chopped spinach or kale

- 1/2 cup diced tomatoes
- 1/4 cup diced red onions
- 1/4 cup sliced mushrooms
- 1/4 cup crumbled feta cheese (optional)
- 1 tablespoon olive oil or avocado oil
- Salt and pepper to taste
- Fresh herbs for garnish (e.g., parsley or basil)

Health Tip: The Healthy Components of the Major Ingredients

Let's explore the wholesome components of the major ingredients in this Veggie-Packed Frittata, providing you with a better understanding of the nutritional benefits it offers:

Eggs: Eggs are a nutritional powerhouse, rich in high-quality protein and essential amino acids. They also provide essential vitamins and minerals such as vitamin B12, vitamin D, choline, and selenium. Including eggs in your breakfast can support muscle maintenance, brain function, and overall health.

Bell Peppers: These colorful gems are abundant in vitamin C, providing immune-boosting benefits and supporting collagen production for healthy skin and joints. Bell peppers also offer antioxidants like beta-carotene, lutein, and zeaxanthin, which promote eye health.

Spinach or Kale: Leafy greens like spinach and kale are nutrient-dense, boasting an array of vitamins A, C, K, and minerals like iron and calcium. Incorporating these greens into your frittata adds powerful antioxidants and supports bone health and immune function.

Tomatoes: Tomatoes are a source of lycopene, a potent antioxidant known for its role in reducing the risk of certain chronic diseases. They also provide vitamin C, potassium, and vitamin K, contributing to heart health and bone health.

Red Onions: Red onions offer a distinct flavor and are rich in antioxidants, particularly quercetin, which may help reduce inflammation and support heart health. They also provide fiber and vitamin C.

Mushrooms: Mushrooms are low in calories and rich in B-vitamins, selenium, and antioxidants. They support immune function, help manage blood sugar levels, and offer a savory umami flavor to the frittata.

Feta Cheese (optional): Feta cheese adds a creamy and tangy element to the frittata. While it's optional, feta provides calcium and protein. If you choose to include it, use it in moderation to keep the sodium content in check.

Fresh Herbs: Garnishing your frittata with fresh herbs like parsley or basil not only adds a burst of flavor but also offers additional nutrients and antioxidants.

Instructions:

Step 1: Preheat your oven to 375°F (190°C) to prepare for baking the frittata.

Step 2: In a large bowl, whisk together the eggs and milk until well combined. Season the egg mixture with a pinch of salt and pepper according to your taste preferences. Set the bowl aside for later use.

Step 3: In an oven-safe skillet, heat the olive oil or avocado oil over medium heat. Add the diced red onions and sauté until they become translucent and fragrant.

Step 4: Add the diced bell peppers and sliced mushrooms to the skillet. Sauté the vegetables for a few minutes until they soften slightly. The combination of colorful veggies will lend an array of nutrients and flavors to the frittata.

Step 5: Stir in the chopped spinach or kale and diced tomatoes. Allow the vegetables to cook for another couple of minutes until the greens wilt and the tomatoes release their juices.

Step 6: Pour the whisked egg mixture evenly over the sautéed vegetables in the skillet. Let the eggs settle into the vegetable mixture, creating a cohesive and flavorsome base for your frittata.

Step 7: If desired, sprinkle crumbled feta cheese over the top of the frittata. The tangy and creamy feta pairs wonderfully with the vibrant vegetables.

Step 8: Transfer the skillet to the preheated oven and bake the frittata for approximately 15-20 minutes or until the eggs are fully set and slightly golden on top.

Step 9: Once the frittata is cooked to perfection, remove it from the oven and let it cool slightly in the skillet.

Step 10: Garnish your Veggie-Packed Frittata with fresh herbs like parsley or basil for an added touch of freshness and aroma.

Step 11: Slice the frittata into wedges and serve warm. The combination of nutritious vegetables and protein-rich eggs makes this dish a satisfying and balanced breakfast option. Enjoy the flavors and textures of this Veggie-Packed

Frittata as you embrace the goodness of a veggie-packed start to your day!

- Wholesome Oatmeal with Fresh Berries

Indulge in a comforting and nutritious bowl of Wholesome Oatmeal with Fresh Berries. This hearty breakfast option is a delightful blend of creamy oats and vibrant berries, providing you with a nourishing start to your day. Let's walk through the steps to create this wholesome and satisfying oatmeal bowl:

Ingredients:
- 1 cup rolled oats
- 2 cups water or milk (dairy or plant-based)
- Pinch of salt
- 1 tablespoon honey or maple syrup (optional, for sweetness)
- 1/2 cup fresh berries (such as blueberries, strawberries, or raspberries)
- 1 tablespoon chia seeds (optional, for added nutrients and texture)

- Nuts or seeds for topping (e.g., sliced almonds, chopped walnuts, or pumpkin seeds)

Health Tip: The Healthy Components of the Major Ingredients

Before we proceed, let's explore the wholesome components of the major ingredients in this Wholesome Oatmeal with Fresh Berries, offering you a dose of nutrition and taste:

Oats: Oats are a fantastic source of complex carbohydrates, providing sustained energy to kickstart your day. They are also rich in soluble fiber, which aids in digestion and helps regulate cholesterol levels. Additionally, oats contain vitamins, minerals, and antioxidants that support overall health.

Fresh Berries: Berries are nutritional powerhouses, brimming with antioxidants, vitamins, and fiber. Blueberries, strawberries, and raspberries are particularly rich in vitamin C, vitamin K, and various phytonutrients, offering numerous health benefits, including improved heart health and cognitive function.

Chia Seeds (optional): Chia seeds are small but mighty. They are loaded with omega-3 fatty acids, fiber, protein, and essential minerals like calcium and magnesium. Including chia seeds in your oatmeal provides a satiating boost of nutrition.

Nuts or Seeds for Topping: Adding nuts or seeds like sliced almonds, chopped walnuts, or pumpkin seeds enhances the texture and taste of the oatmeal. Nuts and seeds offer healthy fats, protein, and additional nutrients, promoting heart health and satiety.

Instructions:

Step 1: In a saucepan, bring the water or milk (dairy or plant-based) to a gentle boil.

Step 2: Add the rolled oats and a pinch of salt to the boiling liquid, stirring continuously.

Step 3: Reduce the heat to medium-low and let the oats simmer for 5-7 minutes, stirring occasionally. The oats will absorb the liquid and soften, creating a creamy and comforting texture.

Step 4: If desired, add honey or maple syrup to sweeten the oatmeal to your taste preferences. You can adjust the sweetness to cater to your individual liking.

Step 5: Remove the saucepan from the heat and let the oatmeal sit for a minute to thicken.

Step 6: In a serving bowl, ladle the warm and creamy oatmeal.

Step 7: Top the oatmeal with an array of fresh berries, such as blueberries, strawberries, or raspberries. The burst of colors will brighten your morning and add a delightful sweetness.

Step 8: Sprinkle chia seeds over the berries, if using, for an extra boost of nutrients and a pleasant crunch.

Step 9: Complete your wholesome creation by adding your favorite nuts or seeds as a topping. The addition of sliced almonds, chopped walnuts, or pumpkin seeds not only elevates the taste but also contributes to a satisfying and nourishing breakfast.

Step 10: Take a moment to savor the delightful blend of flavors and textures in your Wholesome Oatmeal with Fresh Berries. Enjoy the nutritious goodness of oats, the antioxidant-rich sweetness of berries, and the wholesome crunch of nuts or seeds.

Step 11: Embrace the nourishing and comforting qualities of this breakfast bowl as you fuel your body and mind for the day ahead. This Wholesome Oatmeal with Fresh Berries is a delightful way to start your morning on a nutritious and delicious note.

- Chia Seed Pudding with Almond Milk

Savor the delectable and nutrient-packed Chia Seed Pudding with Almond Milk, a delightful and creamy treat that can be enjoyed as a wholesome breakfast or a guilt-free dessert.

Let's dive into the recipe and discover the simple steps to create this delightful chia seed pudding:

Ingredients:
- 1/4 cup chia seeds
- 1 cup unsweetened almond milk (or any milk of your choice)
- 1 tablespoon maple syrup or honey (adjust to your preferred level of sweetness)
- 1/2 teaspoon vanilla extract (optional, for added flavor)
- Fresh fruits for topping (e.g., sliced strawberries, blueberries, or kiwi)
- Nuts or granola for added crunch (optional)

Health Tip: The Healthy Components of the Major Ingredients

Before we proceed, let's explore the nourishing components of the major ingredients in this Chia Seed Pudding with Almond Milk, offering you a delightful balance of taste and nutrition:

Chia Seeds: Chia seeds are nutrient powerhouses, packed with fiber, omega-3 fatty acids, protein, and essential minerals like calcium, magnesium, and phosphorus. They absorb liquid, forming a gel-like texture, making them a perfect base for pudding. Chia seeds also support digestion and satiety.

Almond Milk: Unsweetened almond milk is a creamy and dairy-free alternative to traditional milk. It is low in calories and rich in vitamin E, providing a nourishing base for your chia seed pudding. Almond milk is also suitable for those with lactose intolerance or dairy allergies.

Maple Syrup or Honey: Natural sweeteners like maple syrup or honey add a touch of sweetness to the pudding without the need for refined sugars. Use them in moderation to maintain the balance of flavors and nutrients.

Fresh Fruits: Topping your chia seed pudding with fresh fruits like sliced strawberries, blueberries, or kiwi enhances the sweetness and adds essential vitamins, minerals, and antioxidants to your dessert.

Nuts or Granola: Adding nuts or granola as a topping offers a delightful crunch and an extra dose of protein, healthy fats, and nutrients to your chia seed pudding.

Instructions:

Step 1: In a mixing bowl, combine the chia seeds, unsweetened almond milk, maple syrup or honey, and vanilla extract (if using). Stir well to ensure the chia seeds are evenly distributed.

Step 2: Let the mixture sit for a few minutes, then give it another stir to prevent clumping. Continue to stir every few minutes for the next 15-20 minutes to achieve a smooth and creamy consistency.

Step 3: Once the mixture has thickened, cover the bowl and refrigerate the chia seed pudding for at least 3 hours or overnight. The chia seeds will fully absorb the almond milk, creating a pudding-like texture.

Step 4: Before serving, give the pudding a final stir to ensure a uniform texture.

Step 5: Spoon the Chia Seed Pudding with Almond Milk into serving bowls or glasses.

Step 6: Top your pudding with an array of fresh fruits, such as sliced strawberries, blueberries, or kiwi. The combination of chia seeds and fruit creates a delightful harmony of textures and flavors.

Step 7: If desired, sprinkle nuts or granola on top for added crunch and nutrition. This step is optional, but it adds a pleasant contrast to the creamy pudding.

Step 8: Take a moment to admire the beauty of your Chia Seed Pudding with Almond Milk before diving in!

Step 9: Savor each spoonful of this nourishing and delicious dessert. Enjoy the creamy richness of the chia seeds and almond milk, balanced with the natural sweetness of fresh fruits.

Step 10: Embrace the goodness of this Chia Seed Pudding with Almond Milk as a delightful way to indulge in a guilt-free treat that offers a boost of energy and nutrients. Whether enjoyed for breakfast, as a snack, or as a dessert, this pudding is sure to delight your taste buds and nourish your body with wholesome goodness.

Chapter 3:

Scrumptious Lunches

- Grilled Portobello Mushroom Burger

Treat yourself to a delightful and hearty Grilled Portobello Mushroom Burger, a satisfying lunch option that caters to both vegetarians and burger enthusiasts alike. This scrumptious burger is a delicious twist on the classic, with the meaty and savory portobello mushroom as the star. Let's walk through the steps to create this mouthwatering grilled mushroom burger:

Ingredients:
- 4 large portobello mushrooms, stems removed
- 1/4 cup balsamic vinegar
- 2 tablespoons olive oil
- 2 garlic cloves, minced
- 1 teaspoon dried thyme (or any preferred herbs)

- Salt and pepper to taste
- 4 whole-grain burger buns
- Fresh lettuce leaves
- Sliced tomatoes
- Sliced red onions
- Condiments of your choice (e.g., avocado spread, hummus, or mustard)

Health Tip: The Benefits of Portobello Mushrooms

Before we proceed with the recipe, let's explore the health benefits of portobello mushrooms, making this burger not only delicious but also a nutritious choice:

Rich in Nutrients: Portobello mushrooms are a low-calorie food that provides essential nutrients, including vitamins B3, B5, and B6, as well as minerals like potassium, phosphorus, and selenium. These nutrients play vital roles in various bodily functions.

Source of Antioxidants: Portobello mushrooms contain antioxidants like ergothioneine and selenium, which help combat oxidative stress and protect the cells from damage.

High in Fiber: These mushrooms are an excellent source of dietary fiber, supporting digestive health and promoting a feeling of fullness.

Instructions:

Step 1: In a shallow dish, whisk together the balsamic vinegar, olive oil, minced garlic, dried thyme (or your preferred herbs), and a pinch of salt and pepper to create the marinade.

Step 2: Place the portobello mushrooms in the marinade, ensuring they are well coated. Let the mushrooms marinate for at least 30 minutes to allow the flavors to infuse.

Step 3: Preheat your grill or stovetop grill pan over medium-high heat.

Step 4: While the grill is preheating, prepare the burger buns and toppings. You can lightly toast the buns for added texture and warmth.

Step 5: Grill the marinated portobello mushrooms for approximately 4-5 minutes on each side, or until they become tender and slightly charred. Basting the mushrooms with the remaining marinade during grilling will enhance the flavors.

Step 6: Once the mushrooms are grilled to perfection, remove them from the heat and let them rest for a minute.

Step 7: Assemble your Grilled Portobello Mushroom Burger by placing a grilled mushroom on the bottom half of each bun.

Step 8: Top the mushroom with fresh lettuce leaves, sliced tomatoes, and sliced red onions.

Step 9: Enhance the burger with your choice of condiments, such as avocado spread, hummus, or mustard, to add creaminess and extra flavor.

Step 10: Place the top half of the bun on the condiments to complete your delicious burger.

Step 11: Serve your Grilled Portobello Mushroom Burger with a side of crispy sweet potato fries or a fresh green salad for a balanced and delightful lunch.

Step 12: Take a moment to savor each mouthful of this scrumptious and nutritious burger. Enjoy the hearty and savory taste of the portobello mushroom, perfectly complemented by the fresh and crunchy toppings.

Step 13: Embrace the wholesome goodness of this Grilled Portobello Mushroom Burger as a delectable lunch option that combines great taste and health benefits in one delightful package.

- Lentil and Vegetable Soup

Warm your soul with a comforting bowl of Lentil and Vegetable Soup, a hearty and nutritious lunch option that will keep you energized and satisfied. This delicious soup is a delightful medley of lentils, vibrant vegetables, and flavorful herbs, making it a perfect choice for a wholesome lunch. Let's dive into the recipe and discover the steps to create this nourishing soup:

Ingredients:
- 1 cup dried lentils (green or brown), rinsed and drained
- 6 cups vegetable broth (low-sodium)
- 1 tablespoon olive oil
- 1 large onion, finely chopped
- 2 carrots, diced
- 2 celery stalks, diced
- 2 garlic cloves, minced
- 1 can diced tomatoes (14 ounces), undrained
- 1 teaspoon ground cumin
- 1 teaspoon dried thyme
- 1 bay leaf
- Salt and pepper to taste
- Fresh parsley for garnish (optional)

Health Tip: The Benefits of Lentils and Vegetables

Before we proceed with the recipe, let's explore the health benefits of lentils and vegetables, making this soup not only delicious but also a nutritious choice:

Lentils: Lentils are a fantastic source of plant-based protein and are rich in dietary fiber, promoting a feeling of fullness and supporting digestive health. They are also packed with essential nutrients such as iron, folate, and magnesium.

Vegetables: The combination of onions, carrots, celery, and garlic adds essential vitamins, minerals, and antioxidants to the soup. These vegetables support immune function, heart health, and overall well-being.

Instructions:

Step 1: In a large pot, heat the olive oil over medium heat.

Step 2: Add the chopped onion, diced carrots, and diced celery to the pot. Sauté the vegetables for 4-5 minutes or until they become tender and slightly golden.

Step 3: Stir in the minced garlic and cook for an additional minute until the garlic becomes fragrant.

Step 4: Add the rinsed lentils to the pot, along with the vegetable broth.

Step 5: Stir in the diced tomatoes, including their juice, to enhance the flavor and texture of the soup.

Step 6: Season the soup with ground cumin, dried thyme, bay leaf, salt, and pepper. These herbs and spices will infuse the soup with delightful aromas and flavors.

Step 7: Bring the soup to a boil, then reduce the heat to low. Let the soup simmer for approximately 25-30 minutes or until the lentils are tender and the flavors have melded.

Step 8: While the soup is simmering, take the time to prepare any desired garnish or side dishes.

Step 9: Once the lentils are cooked to perfection, remove the bay leaf from the soup.

Step 10: Ladle the warm and nourishing Lentil and Vegetable Soup into serving bowls.

Step 11: Garnish each bowl with fresh parsley, if desired, to add a pop of color and an herbal note.

Step 12: Enjoy your comforting and wholesome Lentil and Vegetable Soup as a delightful lunch. The combination of protein-rich lentils and nutrient-packed vegetables will keep you feeling satisfied and energized throughout the day.

Step 13: Serve the soup with a side of crusty whole-grain bread or a fresh green salad for a complete and satisfying meal.

Step 14: Take a moment to savor the nourishment and flavors of this hearty soup, knowing that you are treating your body to a nourishing and delicious lunch option.

- Quinoa and Avocado Salad

Treat yourself to a refreshing and wholesome Quinoa and Avocado Salad, a delightful lunch option that combines the nutty goodness of quinoa with the creamy richness of avocados. This salad is a burst of colors and flavors, packed with nutritious ingredients that will keep you feeling nourished and satisfied. Let's dive into the recipe and discover the steps to create this delicious and nutritious salad:

Ingredients:
- 1 cup quinoa, rinsed
- 2 cups water or vegetable broth
- 2 ripe avocados, diced
- 1 cup cherry tomatoes, halved
- 1/2 cucumber, diced
- 1/4 cup red onion, finely chopped
- 1/4 cup fresh cilantro or parsley, chopped
- 1/4 cup crumbled feta cheese (optional)
- 2 tablespoons extra-virgin olive oil
- 1 tablespoon fresh lemon juice
- 1 clove garlic, minced

- Salt and pepper to taste

Health Tip: The Benefits of Quinoa and Avocado

Before we proceed with the recipe, let's explore the health benefits of quinoa and avocados, making this salad not only delicious but also a nutritious choice:

Quinoa: Quinoa is a complete protein source, containing all essential amino acids. It is also rich in fiber, vitamins, and minerals like magnesium and phosphorus, supporting digestion and overall health.

Avocado: Avocados are a great source of heart-healthy monounsaturated fats, which help lower bad cholesterol levels. They are also packed with vitamins, minerals, and antioxidants, promoting skin health and providing a feeling of fullness.

Instructions:

Step 1: In a saucepan, combine the rinsed quinoa and water or vegetable broth. Bring the liquid to a boil over medium-high heat.

Step 2: Reduce the heat to low, cover the saucepan, and let the quinoa simmer for approximately 15-20 minutes or until the quinoa is cooked and the liquid is absorbed. Fluff the quinoa with a fork and set it aside to cool.

Step 3: While the quinoa is cooling, prepare the other ingredients for the salad.

Step 4: In a large mixing bowl, combine the diced avocados, halved cherry tomatoes, diced cucumber, finely chopped red onion, and fresh cilantro or parsley.

Step 5: If desired, add crumbled feta cheese to the salad for an extra burst of flavor and creaminess.

Step 6: In a small bowl, whisk together the extra-virgin olive oil, fresh lemon juice, minced garlic, salt, and pepper to create the dressing.

Step 7: Pour the dressing over the avocado and vegetable mixture, tossing gently to coat the ingredients evenly.

Step 8: Once the quinoa has cooled to room temperature, add it to the salad bowl. The quinoa will add a delightful nutty flavor and provide additional protein and fiber to the salad.

Step 9: Gently toss all the ingredients together until well combined, making sure the dressing is evenly distributed.

Step 10: Take a moment to admire the vibrant colors and fresh ingredients of your Quinoa and Avocado Salad.

Step 11: Serve the salad in individual bowls or on a large platter for a delightful lunch option.

Step 12: Enjoy the refreshing and nutritious combination of quinoa, creamy avocados, and crisp vegetables in every mouthful of this salad.

Step 13: Embrace the wholesome goodness of this Quinoa and Avocado Salad as a satisfying and nourishing lunch that provides a perfect balance of flavors and nutrients.

Step 14: Serve the salad as is or alongside your favorite protein source for a complete and well-rounded meal. Whether enjoyed as a light lunch or a refreshing side dish, this salad is sure to leave you feeling nourished and satisfied.

- Spinach and Chickpea Wrap

Savor the delightful flavors and textures of a Spinach and Chickpea Wrap, a nutritious and satisfying lunch option that celebrates the goodness of plant-based ingredients. This wrap is a wholesome combination of spinach, protein-packed chickpeas, and flavorful seasonings, all wrapped in a soft tortilla. Let's dive into the recipe and create this delectable and easy-to-make wrap:

Ingredients:
- 1 cup cooked chickpeas (canned or cooked from dried)
- 2 cups fresh spinach leaves
- 1/4 cup diced red bell pepper
- 1/4 cup diced cucumber
- 1/4 cup shredded carrots
- 2 tablespoons chopped red onion
- 2 tablespoons chopped fresh parsley or cilantro
- 1 tablespoon lemon juice
- 1 tablespoon olive oil
- 1/2 teaspoon ground cumin
- 1/2 teaspoon paprika
- Salt and pepper to taste
- Whole-grain or gluten-free tortillas

Health Tip: The Benefits of Spinach and Chickpeas

Before we proceed with the recipe, let's explore the health benefits of spinach and chickpeas, making this wrap not only delicious but also a nutritious choice:

Spinach: Spinach is a nutrient-dense leafy green, rich in vitamins A, C, K, and folate. It also provides essential minerals like iron and calcium. Including spinach in your wrap adds a boost of antioxidants and supports bone health.

Chickpeas: Chickpeas, also known as garbanzo beans, are an excellent source of plant-based protein and fiber. They are also rich in folate, iron, phosphorus, and B-vitamins, promoting digestive health and providing sustained energy.

Instructions:

Step 1: In a mixing bowl, combine the cooked chickpeas, fresh spinach leaves, diced red bell pepper, diced cucumber, shredded carrots, chopped red onion, and chopped fresh parsley or cilantro.

Step 2: In a small bowl, whisk together the lemon juice, olive oil, ground cumin, paprika, salt, and pepper to create the dressing.

Step 3: Pour the dressing over the chickpea and vegetable mixture, tossing gently to coat all the ingredients with the flavorful dressing.

Step 4: Taste the mixture and adjust the seasonings, as needed, to suit your taste preferences.

Step 5: Warm the tortillas in a microwave or on a skillet to make them more pliable for wrapping.

Step 6: Spoon the spinach and chickpea filling onto the center of each tortilla, leaving space on the sides for folding.

Step 7: Fold in the sides of the tortilla and then roll it up tightly to form a wrap.

Step 8: Repeat the process to make additional wraps based on the number of servings needed.

Step 9: Take a moment to appreciate the vibrant colors and fresh ingredients in your Spinach and Chickpea Wrap.

Step 10: Serve the wraps as a delightful and portable lunch option, perfect for enjoying at home, work, or on the go.

Step 11: Pair the wraps with a side salad or a serving of fresh fruits for a well-rounded and balanced meal.

Step 12: Enjoy each bite of this Spinach and Chickpea Wrap, savoring the combination of flavors and the satisfying crunch of the vegetables.

Step 13: Embrace the nourishing goodness of this plant-based wrap, knowing that you are treating your taste buds and body to a wholesome and delicious lunch option.

Step 14: Whether you are a fan of plant-based meals or simply seeking a delightful and nutritious lunch, this Spinach and Chickpea

Wrap is sure to become a favorite in your meal repertoire.

Chapter 4:

Delectable Dinners

- Baked Salmon with Lemon-Dill Sauce

Indulge in a mouthwatering and nutritious dinner with Baked Salmon accompanied by a zesty Lemon-Dill Sauce. This delectable dish is not only easy to prepare but also a delightful celebration of flavors that will impress your taste buds and guests alike. Let's dive into the recipe and discover how to create this exquisite dinner:

Ingredients:
- 4 salmon fillets (approximately 6 ounces each), skin-on or skinless
- 2 tablespoons olive oil
- 1 tablespoon fresh lemon juice
- 2 garlic cloves, minced

- 1 teaspoon dried dill (or 1 tablespoon fresh dill, chopped)
- 1/2 teaspoon paprika
- Salt and pepper to taste

For the Lemon-Dill Sauce:
- 1/2 cup plain Greek yogurt (or sour cream for a creamier sauce)
- 1 tablespoon fresh lemon juice
- 1 tablespoon fresh dill, chopped
- 1 teaspoon Dijon mustard
- Salt and pepper to taste

Health Tip: The Benefits of Salmon

Before we proceed with the recipe, let's explore the health benefits of salmon, making this dinner not only delectable but also a nutritious choice:

Salmon: Salmon is an excellent source of omega-3 fatty acids, which are essential for heart health and brain function. It is also rich in high-quality protein, vitamin D, and selenium. Consuming salmon regularly supports overall health and well-being.

Instructions:

Step 1: Preheat your oven to 375°F (190°C) to prepare for baking the salmon.

Step 2: In a small bowl, whisk together the olive oil, fresh lemon juice, minced garlic, dried dill (or fresh dill), paprika, salt, and pepper to create the marinade for the salmon.

Step 3: Place the salmon fillets in a baking dish, arranging them in a single layer.

Step 4: Pour the marinade over the salmon fillets, ensuring they are well coated. Let the salmon marinate for about 15-20 minutes to allow the flavors to infuse.

Step 5: While the salmon is marinating, prepare the Lemon-Dill Sauce by combining the plain Greek yogurt (or sour cream), fresh lemon juice, chopped dill, Dijon mustard, salt, and pepper in a small bowl. Mix well until the sauce is smooth and creamy. Adjust the seasonings to your taste preferences.

Step 6: After marinating, remove the salmon fillets from the baking dish and place them on a lined baking sheet.

Step 7: Bake the salmon in the preheated oven for approximately 15-20 minutes or until the salmon is cooked through and flakes easily with a fork.

Step 8: While the salmon is baking, you can prepare your desired side dishes, such as roasted vegetables or a quinoa salad.

Step 9: Once the salmon is baked to perfection, remove it from the oven and let it rest for a minute.

Step 10: Serve the Baked Salmon with a generous drizzle of the zesty Lemon-Dill Sauce on top of each fillet.

Step 11: Take a moment to appreciate the aroma and presentation of your exquisite dinner.

Step 12: Serve the Baked Salmon with Lemon-Dill Sauce alongside your favorite side dishes for a well-balanced and satisfying dinner.

Step 13: Savor each succulent and flavorful bite of the salmon, relishing the delicate balance of herbs and spices.

Step 14: Embrace the nourishing goodness of this delectable dinner, knowing that you have treated yourself and your loved ones to a delightful and wholesome meal.

Step 15: Whether enjoyed on a special occasion or as a regular dinner option, Baked Salmon with Lemon-Dill Sauce is sure to become a star dish in your culinary repertoire.

- Stir-Fried Tofu with Broccoli and Ginger

Delight in the flavors and textures of a mouthwatering Stir-Fried Tofu with Broccoli and Ginger, a wholesome and plant-based dinner that celebrates the versatility of tofu and the vibrant goodness of broccoli. This delicious stir-fry is a delightful medley of colors and tastes, making it a perfect choice for a satisfying and nutritious dinner. Let's dive into the recipe and discover how to create this delectable stir-fry:

Ingredients:
- 1 block of firm tofu, drained and cubed
- 2 cups broccoli florets
- 1 red bell pepper, thinly sliced
- 2 tablespoons soy sauce (or tamari for a gluten-free option)
- 1 tablespoon hoisin sauce
- 1 tablespoon rice vinegar
- 1 tablespoon sesame oil
- 1 tablespoon fresh ginger, minced
- 2 garlic cloves, minced
- 2 green onions, sliced (white and green parts separated)
- 1 tablespoon vegetable oil for stir-frying
- Sesame seeds for garnish (optional)
- Cooked brown rice or quinoa for serving

Health Tip: The Benefits of Tofu and Broccoli

Before we proceed with the recipe, let's explore the health benefits of tofu and broccoli, making this stir-fry not only delightful but also a nutritious choice:

Tofu: Tofu is an excellent source of plant-based protein, making it a valuable component of vegetarian and vegan diets. It is also rich in calcium, iron, and various essential vitamins and minerals. Tofu supports bone health, muscle function, and overall well-being.

Broccoli: Broccoli is a cruciferous vegetable that is packed with vitamins, minerals, and antioxidants. It is particularly rich in vitamin C, vitamin K, and folate. Broccoli supports immune function, heart health, and healthy digestion.

Instructions:
Step 1: In a small bowl, combine the soy sauce, hoisin sauce, rice vinegar, and sesame oil to create the stir-fry sauce. Set the sauce aside.

Step 2: In a wok or large skillet, heat the vegetable oil over medium-high heat.

Step 3: Add the cubed tofu to the hot oil and stir-fry for 4-5 minutes, or until the tofu becomes slightly golden and crispy on the edges.

Step 4: Add the minced ginger and garlic to the tofu, continuing to stir-fry for another minute until the aroma is released.

Step 5: Toss in the sliced white parts of the green onions, as well as the broccoli florets and red bell pepper. Stir-fry for an additional 3-4 minutes until the vegetables are slightly tender but still crisp.

Step 6: Pour the prepared stir-fry sauce over the tofu and vegetables, stirring to coat them evenly.

Step 7: Continue to stir-fry for another 2-3 minutes, allowing the sauce to thicken and infuse the flavors into the tofu and vegetables.

Step 8: Once the tofu and vegetables are coated in the flavorful sauce and heated through, remove the stir-fry from the heat.

Step 9: Garnish the Stir-Fried Tofu with Broccoli and Ginger with the sliced green parts of the green onions and a sprinkle of sesame seeds, if desired.

Step 10: Serve the stir-fry over a bed of cooked brown rice or quinoa for a complete and satisfying meal.

Step 11: Take a moment to appreciate the beautiful colors and enticing aromas of your Stir-Fried Tofu with Broccoli and Ginger.

Step 12: Enjoy each mouthful of this wholesome and flavorful stir-fry, relishing the tender tofu, crunchy vegetables, and aromatic ginger.

Step 13: Embrace the nourishing goodness of this plant-based dinner, knowing that you have treated yourself to a delightful and nutrient-packed meal.

Step 14: Whether you are following a vegetarian lifestyle or simply seeking a delicious and nutritious dinner, Stir-Fried Tofu with Broccoli and Ginger is sure to become a favorite in your dinner rotation.

- Stuffed Bell Peppers with Quinoa and Spinach

Indulge in a delightful and wholesome dinner with Stuffed Bell Peppers filled with the goodness of quinoa and spinach. This delicious and colorful dish is not only a feast for the eyes but also a nutritious and satisfying meal. Let's dive into the recipe and discover how to create these flavorful stuffed bell peppers:

Ingredients:
- 4 large bell peppers (any color), tops removed and seeds removed
- 1 cup cooked quinoa

- 1 cup fresh spinach, chopped
- 1 can (14 ounces) diced tomatoes, drained
- 1 can (14 ounces) black beans, drained and rinsed
- 1/2 cup diced red onion
- 2 garlic cloves, minced
- 1 teaspoon ground cumin
- 1 teaspoon chili powder
- 1/2 teaspoon paprika
- Salt and pepper to taste
- 1 cup shredded mozzarella or cheddar cheese (optional, for topping)

Health Tip: The Benefits of Bell Peppers, Quinoa, and Spinach

Before we proceed with the recipe, let's explore the health benefits of bell peppers, quinoa, and spinach, making this dish not only delicious but also a nutritious choice:

Bell Peppers: Bell peppers are rich in vitamin C, vitamin A, and antioxidants, supporting immune function and promoting healthy skin. They add a vibrant touch to the dish while providing essential nutrients.

Quinoa: Quinoa is a nutrient-dense grain that is gluten-free and packed with protein, fiber, vitamins, and minerals. It supports digestive health and provides sustained energy.

Spinach: Spinach is a leafy green vegetable that is rich in iron, calcium, and vitamins A and K. It promotes bone health and supports overall well-being.

Instructions:

Step 1: Preheat your oven to 375°F (190°C) to prepare for baking the stuffed bell peppers.

Step 2: In a large mixing bowl, combine the cooked quinoa, chopped fresh spinach, diced tomatoes, black beans, diced red onion, minced garlic, ground cumin, chili powder, paprika, salt, and pepper. Mix well to ensure all the ingredients are evenly distributed.

Step 3: Stuff each bell pepper with the quinoa and spinach mixture, pressing down gently to fill them completely.

Step 4: Place the stuffed bell peppers in a baking dish, ensuring they are standing upright and are stable.

Step 5: If using cheese, sprinkle the shredded mozzarella or cheddar on top of each stuffed bell pepper.

Step 6: Cover the baking dish with aluminum foil, creating a tent to prevent the cheese from sticking to it.

Step 7: Bake the stuffed bell peppers in the preheated oven for approximately 25-30 minutes or until the peppers are tender and the filling is heated through.

Step 8: Remove the foil during the last 5 minutes of baking to allow the cheese to melt and turn slightly golden.

Step 9: Once the stuffed bell peppers are baked to perfection, remove them from the oven and let them cool slightly.

Step 10: Take a moment to admire the vibrant colors and inviting aromas of your Stuffed Bell Peppers with Quinoa and Spinach.

Step 11: Serve the stuffed bell peppers as a delightful and nutritious dinner option.

Step 12: Enjoy each mouthful of this flavorful and satisfying dish, savoring the combination of tender bell peppers and the hearty quinoa and spinach filling.

Step 13: Embrace the nourishing goodness of this dinner, knowing that you have treated yourself and your loved ones to a wholesome and delicious meal.

Step 14: Whether you are following a vegetarian lifestyle or simply seeking a delightful and nutritious dinner, Stuffed Bell Peppers with Quinoa and Spinach is sure to become a favorite in your dinner rotation.

- Eggplant Parmesan with Cashew Cheese

Indulge in the deliciousness of Eggplant Parmesan with a twist—creamy and dairy-free Cashew Cheese. This flavorful and comforting dish is a delightful plant-based version of the classic Italian favorite. Let's dive into the recipe and discover how to create this delectable Eggplant Parmesan with Cashew Cheese:

Ingredients:
- 2 large eggplants, sliced into 1/2-inch rounds
- 1 cup whole wheat bread crumbs (or gluten-free bread crumbs for a gluten-free option)
- 1/2 cup almond flour (or any preferred flour)
- 1 teaspoon dried oregano
- 1 teaspoon dried basil
- 1/2 teaspoon garlic powder
- Salt and pepper to taste
- 2 cups marinara sauce (store-bought or homemade)
- Fresh basil leaves for garnish

For the Cashew Cheese:
- 1 cup raw cashews, soaked in water for 2-4 hours and drained
- 1/4 cup nutritional yeast
- 2 tablespoons fresh lemon juice
- 1 tablespoon apple cider vinegar
- 1 clove garlic
- 1/2 cup water (adjust for desired consistency)
- Salt and pepper to taste

Health Tip: The Benefits of Eggplant and Cashews

Before we proceed with the recipe, let's explore the health benefits of eggplant and cashews, making this dish not only delicious but also a nutritious choice:

Eggplant: Eggplant is low in calories and high in fiber, making it a great choice for those looking to manage their weight. It is also rich in antioxidants, particularly nasunin, which supports brain health.

Cashews: Cashews are a good source of healthy fats, protein, and various minerals like magnesium and zinc. They promote heart health and provide sustained energy.

Instructions:

Step 1: Preheat your oven to 375°F (190°C) to prepare for baking the Eggplant Parmesan.

Step 2: In a shallow bowl, combine the whole wheat bread crumbs (or gluten-free bread crumbs), almond flour (or any preferred flour), dried oregano, dried basil, garlic powder, salt, and pepper to create the breading mixture.

Step 3: Dip each eggplant slice into the breading mixture, ensuring they are well coated on both sides. Place the coated eggplant slices on a baking sheet lined with parchment paper.

Step 4: Bake the eggplant slices in the preheated oven for approximately 20-25 minutes or until they become golden and tender. Flip the slices halfway through baking for even cooking.

Step 5: While the eggplant is baking, prepare the Cashew Cheese. In a high-speed blender or food processor, blend the soaked and drained cashews, nutritional yeast, fresh lemon juice, apple cider vinegar, garlic, water, salt, and pepper until smooth and creamy. Adjust the water as needed to achieve your desired consistency.

Step 6: In a baking dish, spread a thin layer of marinara sauce at the bottom.

Step 7: Once the eggplant slices are baked to perfection, remove them from the oven.

Step 8: Place a layer of the baked eggplant slices on top of the marinara sauce in the baking dish.

Step 9: Spread a generous amount of Cashew Cheese on top of the eggplant slices.

Step 10: Repeat the process of layering the eggplant slices and Cashew Cheese until all the eggplant slices are used up.

Step 11: Finish by spreading the remaining marinara sauce over the top layer of the Eggplant Parmesan.

Step 12: Bake the assembled Eggplant Parmesan in the oven for an additional 15-20 minutes or until it becomes bubbly and the flavors meld together.

Step 13: Once the Eggplant Parmesan is baked to perfection, remove it from the oven and let it cool slightly.

Step 14: Garnish the dish with fresh basil leaves for a pop of color and an herbal note.

Step 15: Serve the Eggplant Parmesan with Cashew Cheese as a delightful and satisfying dinner option.

Step 16: Enjoy each mouthful of this creamy, flavorful, and wholesome Eggplant Parmesan, savoring the combination of tender eggplant and the luscious Cashew Cheese.

Step 17: Embrace the nourishing goodness of this dairy-free version of a classic favorite, knowing that you have treated yourself and your loved ones to a delightful and plant-powered meal.

Step 18: Whether you are following a plant-based lifestyle or simply seeking a delicious and nutritious dinner, Eggplant Parmesan with Cashew Cheese is sure to become a new favorite in your culinary repertoire.

Chapter 5:

Satisfying Snacks

- Rice Cakes with Hummus and Cucumber Slices

Treat yourself to a delightful and satisfying snack with Rice Cakes topped with creamy Hummus and refreshing Cucumber Slices. This wholesome and light snack is perfect for those mid-day cravings or as a quick pick-me-up between meals. Let's dive into the recipe and discover how to create this delicious and nutritious snack:

Ingredients:
- Rice cakes (plain or flavored, as per preference)
- Hummus (store-bought or homemade)
- 1 cucumber, thinly sliced
- Fresh dill or parsley for garnish (optional)

Health Tip: The Benefits of Rice Cakes, Hummus, and Cucumbers

Before we proceed with the recipe, let's explore the health benefits of rice cakes, hummus, and cucumbers, making this snack not only delightful but also a nutritious choice:

Rice Cakes: Rice cakes are a low-calorie and gluten-free snack option. They provide a crunchy texture without the added fats and oils, making them a light and satisfying choice.

Hummus: Hummus is made from chickpeas, which are rich in protein, fiber, and various vitamins and minerals. It is also a good source of healthy fats from tahini (sesame seed paste). Hummus supports heart health and provides sustained energy.

Cucumbers: Cucumbers are hydrating and low in calories, making them a refreshing and guilt-free snack. They are rich in vitamins A and K, as well as antioxidants, supporting skin health and promoting hydration.

Instructions:

Step 1: Arrange the rice cakes on a plate or serving platter.

Step 2: Using a spoon or a knife, spread a generous amount of hummus on each rice cake, creating a creamy and flavorful base for the snack.

Step 3: Top each rice cake with thin slices of fresh cucumber. The cool and crisp cucumber slices will add a refreshing and hydrating element to the snack.

Step 4: If desired, garnish the Rice Cakes with Hummus and Cucumber Slices with fresh dill or parsley, adding a pop of herbal flavor and visual appeal.

Step 5: Take a moment to appreciate the colorful and inviting presentation of your satisfying snack.

Step 6: Serve the Rice Cakes with Hummus and Cucumber Slices as a delightful and nutritious snack option.

Step 7: Enjoy each crunchy and creamy bite of this wholesome and light snack, relishing the combination of rice cakes, creamy hummus, and refreshing cucumbers.

Step 8: Embrace the nourishing goodness of this satisfying snack, knowing that you have treated yourself to a delightful and nutritious pick-me-up.

Step 9: Whether enjoyed as a quick snack at home, at work, or on the go, Rice Cakes with Hummus and Cucumber Slices are sure to become your go-to choice for a satisfying and wholesome munch.

Step 10: Feel free to customize this snack by adding your favorite toppings or experimenting with different flavors of rice cakes and hummus. The possibilities are endless, and you can create a snack that perfectly suits your taste preferences.

Step 11: Stay fueled and energized throughout the day with this delightful and nutritious snack option. Whether you need a quick bite before a workout or a tasty treat to satisfy your cravings, Rice Cakes with Hummus and Cucumber Slices have got you covered.

- Trail Mix with Nuts and Dried Fruits

Indulge in a delicious and energizing Trail Mix, packed with a delightful combination of nuts and dried fruits. This wholesome and portable snack is perfect for outdoor adventures, busy days, or anytime you need a quick and nutritious boost. Let's dive into the recipe and discover how to create this delightful Trail Mix with Nuts and Dried Fruits:

Ingredients:
- 1 cup raw almonds
- 1 cup raw cashews
- 1 cup raw walnuts

- 1 cup dried cranberries
- 1 cup dried apricots, chopped
- 1/2 cup pumpkin seeds
- 1/2 cup sunflower seeds
- 1/2 cup coconut flakes (unsweetened)
- 1 teaspoon ground cinnamon (optional)

Health Tip: The Benefits of Nuts and Dried Fruits

Before we proceed with the recipe, let's explore the health benefits of nuts and dried fruits, making this Trail Mix not only delicious but also a nutritious choice:

Nuts: Nuts are a rich source of healthy fats, protein, fiber, vitamins, and minerals. They provide sustained energy and support heart health. Almonds, cashews, and walnuts, in particular, are known for their unique nutrient profiles and numerous health benefits.

Dried Fruits: Dried fruits are concentrated sources of vitamins, minerals, and antioxidants. They provide natural sweetness to the Trail Mix without the need for added sugars. Dried cranberries and apricots add a burst of flavor and texture to the mix.

Instructions:

Step 1: In a large mixing bowl, combine the raw almonds, cashews, walnuts, dried cranberries, dried apricots, pumpkin seeds, sunflower seeds, and coconut flakes.

Step 2: If desired, sprinkle ground cinnamon over the mixture for added warmth and flavor. Cinnamon pairs wonderfully with the nuts and dried fruits, creating a delightful aroma and taste.

Step 3: Gently toss the ingredients together, ensuring the nuts and dried fruits are evenly distributed throughout the Trail Mix.

Step 4: Take a moment to appreciate the colorful and textured blend of nuts and dried fruits in your Trail Mix.

Step 5: Store the Trail Mix in an airtight container or individual snack-sized bags for easy and portable snacking.

Step 6: Carry the Trail Mix with you on your outdoor adventures, pack it in your lunchbox for a quick and nutritious treat, or keep a stash at your desk for those busy workdays.

Step 7: Enjoy each handful of this energizing and flavorful Trail Mix, savoring the combination of crunchy nuts and chewy dried fruits.

Step 8: Embrace the nourishing goodness of this wholesome and convenient snack, knowing that you have treated yourself to a delightful and nutrient-packed pick-me-up.

Step 9: Feel free to customize this Trail Mix by adding your favorite nuts, seeds, or dried fruits. You can create different variations to suit your taste preferences and dietary needs.

Step 10: Stay fueled and satisfied throughout the day with this delightful and nutritious Trail

Mix. Whether you are hiking in nature, powering through a busy day, or simply craving a tasty snack, Trail Mix with Nuts and Dried Fruits is the perfect choice to keep you going strong.

- Guacamole with Veggie Sticks

Indulge in the creamy and flavorful goodness of Guacamole, paired with an assortment of fresh Veggie Sticks for a nutritious and satisfying snack. This delightful combination offers a burst of colors, textures, and flavors, making it a perfect choice for a guilt-free treat or a party appetizer. Let's dive into the recipe and discover how to create this delicious Guacamole with Veggie Sticks:

Ingredients:
- 3 ripe avocados
- 1 small red onion, finely diced
- 1 ripe tomato, diced

- 1 jalapeño pepper, seeds removed and finely diced (optional, for heat)
- 1/4 cup fresh cilantro, chopped
- 1-2 tablespoons fresh lime juice
- 1 garlic clove, minced
- Salt and pepper to taste
- Assorted Veggie Sticks (carrots, cucumber, bell peppers, celery, etc.) for dipping

Health Tip: The Benefits of Avocado and Fresh Veggies

Before we proceed with the recipe, let's explore the health benefits of avocados and fresh veggies, making this Guacamole with Veggie Sticks not only delicious but also a nutritious choice:

Avocado: Avocados are rich in heart-healthy monounsaturated fats, which support good cholesterol levels and overall heart health. They are also a good source of fiber, potassium, vitamins C and K, and various antioxidants.

Fresh Veggies: Fresh vegetables are low in calories and high in fiber, vitamins, minerals, and antioxidants. They support digestive health, immune function, and overall well-being.

Instructions:

Step 1: Cut the avocados in half, remove the pits, and scoop out the flesh into a medium-sized bowl.

Step 2: Using a fork, mash the avocado until it reaches your desired consistency. Some people prefer a chunky texture, while others like it smoother.

Step 3: Add the finely diced red onion, diced tomato, and chopped fresh cilantro to the mashed avocado.

Step 4: If you prefer a spicy guacamole, add the finely diced jalapeño pepper to the mixture. Adjust the amount of jalapeño according to your spice tolerance.

Step 5: Squeeze one to two tablespoons of fresh lime juice over the guacamole mixture.

Lime juice not only adds a tangy flavor but also helps prevent the avocados from browning.

Step 6: Add the minced garlic to the guacamole for an extra burst of flavor.

Step 7: Season the guacamole with salt and pepper to taste. Adjust the seasoning as needed to suit your preferences.

Step 8: Gently stir all the ingredients together until well combined.

Step 9: Take a moment to appreciate the vibrant colors and inviting aroma of your freshly made guacamole.

Step 10: Prepare an assortment of Veggie Sticks by slicing carrots, cucumber, bell peppers, celery, or any other favorite veggies into strips or rounds for dipping.

Step 11: Arrange the Veggie Sticks on a serving platter alongside the bowl of guacamole.

Step 12: Serve the Guacamole with Veggie Sticks as a delightful and nutritious snack or appetizer.

Step 13: Enjoy each dip of your Veggie Sticks into the creamy and flavorful guacamole, savoring the combination of fresh vegetables and the rich taste of avocados.

Step 14: Embrace the nourishing goodness of this wholesome and satisfying snack, knowing that you have treated yourself to a delicious and nutrient-packed treat.

Step 15: Whether you are hosting a party, enjoying a movie night at home, or simply craving a tasty and healthy snack, Guacamole with Veggie Sticks is the perfect choice to satisfy your taste buds and nourish your body.

- Baked Kale Chips

Delight in the crispy and nutritious goodness of Baked Kale Chips—a guilt-free snack that combines the earthy flavors of kale with a delightful crunch. These homemade chips are not only a delicious treat but also a great way to enjoy the health benefits of kale. Let's dive into the recipe and discover how to create these delectable Baked Kale Chips:

Ingredients:
- 1 bunch of fresh kale (about 8-10 large leaves)
- 1 tablespoon olive oil
- 1 teaspoon garlic powder
- 1 teaspoon paprika
- 1/2 teaspoon salt (adjust to taste)

Health Tip: The Benefits of Kale

Before we proceed with the recipe, let's explore the health benefits of kale, making these Baked Kale Chips not only delicious but also a nutritious choice:

Kale: Kale is a nutrient powerhouse, packed with vitamins A, C, and K, as well as calcium, iron, and antioxidants. It supports bone health, immune function, and overall well-being.

Instructions:

Step 1: Preheat your oven to 350°F (175°C) to prepare for baking the kale chips.

Step 2: Wash the kale leaves thoroughly under cold water and pat them dry with a kitchen towel or paper towels.

Step 3: Remove the tough stems from the kale leaves and tear the leaves into bite-sized pieces. Discard the stems or save them for other recipes like smoothies or vegetable broth.

Step 4: In a large mixing bowl, drizzle the torn kale leaves with olive oil. Use clean hands to massage the oil into the leaves, ensuring they are evenly coated.

Step 5: Sprinkle the garlic powder, paprika, and salt over the kale leaves, tossing them gently to ensure the seasonings are evenly distributed.

Step 6: Line a baking sheet with parchment paper or a silicone baking mat.

Step 7: Arrange the seasoned kale leaves in a single layer on the prepared baking sheet. Avoid crowding the leaves to ensure even baking and crispiness.

Step 8: Place the baking sheet in the preheated oven and bake the kale chips for approximately 10-15 minutes or until the edges of the leaves become crispy and slightly browned. Keep a close eye on them, as they can burn quickly.

Step 9: Remove the baking sheet from the oven and let the kale chips cool for a few minutes. As they cool, they will become even crispier.

Step 10: Take a moment to appreciate the vibrant green color and enticing aroma of your freshly baked kale chips.

Step 11: Transfer the Baked Kale Chips to a serving bowl or plate.

Step 12: Serve the kale chips as a delightful and nutritious snack or appetizer.

Step 13: Enjoy each crispy bite of your Baked Kale Chips, savoring the earthy and slightly savory flavor.

Step 14: Embrace the nourishing goodness of this guilt-free and wholesome snack, knowing that you have treated yourself to a delicious and nutrient-packed treat.

Step 15: Whether you are seeking a healthier alternative to traditional potato chips or simply craving a tasty and nutrient-dense snack, Baked Kale Chips are the perfect choice to satisfy your cravings and nourish your body.

Chapter 6:

Divine Desserts

- Coconut Chia Seed Pudding

Indulge in the creamy and luscious Coconut Chia Seed Pudding—a divine dessert that brings together the goodness of chia seeds and the delightful flavor of coconut. This dairy-free and naturally sweetened treat is not only scrumptious but also a guilt-free way to satisfy your sweet tooth. Let's dive into the recipe and discover how to create this delectable Coconut Chia Seed Pudding:

Ingredients:
- 1/4 cup chia seeds
- 1 cup coconut milk (canned or homemade)
- 1 tablespoon pure maple syrup (or any preferred sweetener)
- 1/2 teaspoon pure vanilla extract
- Fresh berries and shredded coconut for garnish (optional)

Health Tip: The Benefits of Chia Seeds and Coconut Milk

Before we proceed with the recipe, let's explore the health benefits of chia seeds and coconut milk, making this Coconut Chia Seed Pudding not only delicious but also a nutritious choice:

Chia Seeds: Chia seeds are a rich source of omega-3 fatty acids, fiber, protein, and various minerals. They support digestive health, heart health, and provide sustained energy.

Coconut Milk: Coconut milk is a dairy-free alternative to traditional milk, rich in healthy fats, vitamins C and E, and minerals such as potassium and magnesium. It promotes skin health, supports the immune system, and adds a delightful coconut flavor to the pudding.

Instructions:

Step 1: In a medium-sized bowl, combine the chia seeds, coconut milk, pure maple syrup, and pure vanilla extract.

Step 2: Stir the ingredients together until well combined.

Step 3: Cover the bowl and refrigerate the mixture for at least 4 hours or preferably overnight. This allows the chia seeds to absorb the liquid and create a creamy and pudding-like consistency.

Step 4: After refrigeration, take the Coconut Chia Seed Pudding out of the refrigerator and give it a good stir. You can add more coconut milk if you prefer a thinner consistency.

Step 5: Take a moment to appreciate the rich and velvety texture of your Coconut Chia Seed Pudding.

Step 6: If desired, garnish the pudding with fresh berries and shredded coconut for a burst of color and an extra touch of tropical sweetness.

Step 7: Serve the Coconut Chia Seed Pudding in individual dessert bowls or glasses.

Step 8: Enjoy each spoonful of this creamy and naturally sweetened dessert, relishing the combination of chia seeds and the delectable coconut flavor.

Step 9: Embrace the divine goodness of this guilt-free and satisfying dessert, knowing that you have treated yourself to a wholesome and delightful sweet treat.

Step 10: Whether you are ending a special dinner with a light and indulgent dessert or simply craving a nourishing and delicious after-meal delight, Coconut Chia Seed Pudding is the perfect choice to satisfy your sweet cravings while nourishing your body.

Step 11: Feel free to customize this dessert by adding your favorite toppings or incorporating other flavors such as cocoa powder, almond extract, or a sprinkle of cinnamon. The possibilities are endless, and you can create a chia seed pudding that perfectly suits your taste preferences.

- Mixed Berry Parfait with Greek Yogurt

Savor the delightful combination of tangy Greek yogurt and the natural sweetness of mixed berries in this refreshing Mixed Berry Parfait. This parfait not only tastes heavenly but also provides a generous dose of protein and antioxidants, making it a guilt-free and satisfying dessert option. Let's dive into the recipe and discover how to create this luscious Mixed Berry Parfait with Greek Yogurt:

Ingredients:
- 1 cup Greek yogurt (plain or flavored, as per preference)
- 1 cup mixed berries (strawberries, blueberries, raspberries, or any favorite berries)
- 2 tablespoons honey or pure maple syrup (adjust to taste)
- 1/4 cup granola (store-bought or homemade) for added crunch

Health Tip: The Benefits of Greek Yogurt and Mixed Berries

Before we proceed with the recipe, let's explore the health benefits of Greek yogurt and mixed berries, making this Mixed Berry Parfait with Greek Yogurt not only delicious but also a nutritious choice:

Greek Yogurt: Greek yogurt is a protein-packed dairy product, known for its creamy texture and probiotic benefits. It supports gut health, provides essential nutrients, and keeps you feeling full and satisfied.

Mixed Berries: Mixed berries, such as strawberries, blueberries, and raspberries, are rich in antioxidants, vitamins, and fiber. They support brain health, immune function, and heart health.

Instructions:

Step 1: Wash the mixed berries under cold water and pat them dry with a paper towel. If using strawberries, remove the stems and slice them into bite-sized pieces.

Step 2: In a small bowl, drizzle honey or pure maple syrup over the mixed berries and gently toss them to coat. Adjust the sweetness according to your taste preferences.

Step 3: In a separate bowl or glass, layer the Greek yogurt and the sweetened mixed berries.

Step 4: Take a moment to appreciate the vibrant colors and enticing aroma of your beautifully layered Mixed Berry Parfait.

Step 5: Top the parfait with granola for a delightful crunch and added texture.

Step 6: Serve the Mixed Berry Parfait with Greek Yogurt as a refreshing and nourishing dessert or even as a delightful breakfast option.

Step 7: Enjoy each spoonful of this creamy and fruity parfait, savoring the combination of tangy Greek yogurt and the natural sweetness of the mixed berries.

Step 8: Embrace the guilt-free indulgence of this wholesome and satisfying dessert, knowing that you have treated yourself to a delightful and nutrient-packed treat.

Step 9: Whether you are entertaining guests or simply enjoying a moment of self-care, Mixed Berry Parfait with Greek Yogurt is the perfect choice to please your taste buds and nourish your body.

Step 10: Feel free to get creative with this parfait by adding additional layers of nuts, seeds, or other fruits. You can also drizzle a bit of melted dark chocolate for an indulgent twist.

Step 11: Take the time to relish each bite of your Mixed Berry Parfait, appreciating the harmonious blend of flavors and textures that create a truly delightful dessert experience.

- Dark Chocolate Avocado Mousse

Indulge in the rich and velvety goodness of Dark Chocolate Avocado Mousse—a decadent dessert that combines the creaminess of avocados with the luxurious taste of dark chocolate. This delightful mousse is not only a delectable treat but also a healthier alternative to traditional chocolate mousse. Let's dive into the recipe and discover how to create this luscious Dark Chocolate Avocado Mousse:

Ingredients:
- 2 ripe avocados
- 1/4 cup unsweetened cocoa powder
- 1/4 cup pure maple syrup or agave nectar (adjust to taste)
- 1/4 cup almond milk (or any preferred milk)
- 1 teaspoon pure vanilla extract
- A pinch of salt
- Dark chocolate shavings or cocoa powder for garnish (optional)

Health Tip: The Benefits of Avocados and Dark Chocolate

Before we proceed with the recipe, let's explore the health benefits of avocados and dark chocolate, making this Dark Chocolate Avocado Mousse not only delicious but also a nutritious choice:

Avocados: Avocados are a rich source of heart-healthy monounsaturated fats, vitamins C, E, and K, and various minerals. They promote skin health, support brain function, and contribute to overall well-being.

Dark Chocolate: Dark chocolate, with a high cocoa content, is loaded with antioxidants and beneficial compounds. It can improve heart health, enhance mood, and provide a touch of indulgence without excessive added sugars.

Instructions:

Step 1: Cut the avocados in half, remove the pits, and scoop out the flesh into a blender or food processor.

Step 2: Add the unsweetened cocoa powder, pure maple syrup or agave nectar, almond milk, pure vanilla extract, and a pinch of salt to the blender or food processor.

Step 3: Blend the ingredients until the mixture becomes smooth and creamy. Scrape down the sides as needed to ensure everything is well combined.

Step 4: Taste the Dark Chocolate Avocado Mousse and adjust the sweetness with additional maple syrup or agave nectar if desired.

Step 5: Take a moment to appreciate the luscious texture and rich aroma of your freshly made mousse.

Step 6: If desired, garnish the mousse with dark chocolate shavings or a light dusting of cocoa powder for an elegant finishing touch.

Step 7: Transfer the Dark Chocolate Avocado Mousse to individual dessert bowls or glasses.

Step 8: Serve the mousse as a luxurious and delightful dessert option.

Step 9: Enjoy each spoonful of this creamy and chocolatey delight, savoring the combination of avocados and the indulgence of dark chocolate.

Step 10: Embrace the guilt-free indulgence of this healthier dessert, knowing that you have treated yourself to a delicious and nutrient-packed treat.

Step 11: Whether you are celebrating a special occasion or simply seeking a comforting and satisfying dessert, Dark Chocolate Avocado Mousse is the perfect choice to satisfy your cravings while nourishing your body.

Step 12: Feel free to get creative with this mousse by adding a sprinkle of sea salt, a dollop of whipped coconut cream, or a handful of fresh berries on top.

Step 13: Take the time to savor each spoonful of your Dark Chocolate Avocado Mousse, cherishing the velvety and chocolatey goodness that creates a truly indulgent dessert experience.

- Almond Flour Banana Bread

Enjoy the delightful aroma and comforting taste of Almond Flour Banana Bread—a moist and flavorful treat that combines the sweetness of ripe bananas with the nutty goodness of almond flour. This gluten-free and healthier version of classic banana bread will surely become a favorite in your household. Let's dive into the recipe and discover how to create this scrumptious Almond Flour Banana Bread:

Ingredients:
- 3 ripe bananas, mashed
- 3 large eggs
- 1/4 cup coconut oil, melted (or any preferred oil)
- 1 teaspoon pure vanilla extract
- 2 cups almond flour

- 1/4 cup coconut sugar (or any preferred sweetener)
- 1 teaspoon baking powder
- 1/2 teaspoon baking soda
- 1/2 teaspoon ground cinnamon
- A pinch of salt
- Chopped nuts or dark chocolate chips for added texture (optional)

Health Tip: The Benefits of Almond Flour and Ripe Bananas

Before we proceed with the recipe, let's explore the health benefits of almond flour and ripe bananas, making this Almond Flour Banana Bread not only delicious but also a nutritious choice:

Almond Flour: Almond flour is a gluten-free alternative to wheat flour, rich in healthy fats, protein, and vitamins. It supports heart health, provides sustained energy, and adds a delightful nutty flavor to the banana bread.

Ripe Bananas: Ripe bananas are a great source of vitamins and minerals, particularly potassium and vitamin B6. They are a natural sweetener, allowing you to reduce the amount of added sugars in the recipe.

Instructions:

Step 1: Preheat your oven to 350°F (175°C) and grease a standard-sized loaf pan with a little coconut oil or line it with parchment paper.

Step 2: In a large mixing bowl, mash the ripe bananas using a fork until smooth and creamy.

Step 3: Add the eggs, melted coconut oil, and pure vanilla extract to the mashed bananas, and whisk everything together until well combined.

Step 4: In a separate bowl, combine the almond flour, coconut sugar, baking powder, baking soda, ground cinnamon, and a pinch of salt.

Step 5: Gradually add the dry ingredients to the wet ingredients, stirring until a smooth batter forms. Be careful not to overmix.

Step 6: If desired, fold in chopped nuts or dark chocolate chips to the batter, adding an extra layer of texture and flavor.

Step 7: Pour the batter into the greased or lined loaf pan, spreading it evenly.

Step 8: Take a moment to appreciate the enticing aroma of your freshly prepared Almond Flour Banana Bread.

Step 9: Bake the banana bread in the preheated oven for approximately 45-55 minutes or until a toothpick inserted into the center comes out clean.

Step 10: Remove the pan from the oven and let the banana bread cool in the pan for about 10 minutes.

Step 11: Carefully transfer the banana bread to a wire rack to cool completely.

Step 12: Once cooled, slice the Almond Flour Banana Bread into thick, moist, and delicious slices.

Step 13: Serve the banana bread as a delightful and healthier treat, perfect for breakfast, snack time, or even as a dessert option.

Step 14: Enjoy each bite of this moist and nutty banana bread, savoring the combination of ripe bananas and the richness of almond flour.

Step 15: Embrace the guilt-free indulgence of this gluten-free and wholesome banana bread, knowing that you have treated yourself to a delicious and nourishing treat.

Step 16: Whether enjoyed on its own or with a spread of nut butter or jam, Almond Flour Banana Bread is the perfect choice to bring warmth and comfort to any occasion.

Part 2: A-Negative

Introduction

- Understanding the Blood Type Diet for A-Negative

Welcome to the second part of our cookbook, where we will delve into the fascinating world of the Blood Type Diet specifically tailored for individuals with A-Negative blood type. In this section, we will explore how your blood type influences your body's unique nutritional needs and how following a diet aligned with your blood type can promote optimal health and well-being.

Discovering Your Blood Type:

Before embarking on the journey of the Blood Type Diet, it is essential to know your blood type accurately. If you are unsure of your blood type, we recommend consulting with a healthcare professional or visiting a nearby clinic for a blood test. Knowing your blood type will be the foundation for customizing your dietary choices and embracing a healthier lifestyle.

The Blood Type Diet: A-Negative Perspective:

The Blood Type Diet, introduced by naturopathic physician Dr. Peter J. D'Adamo, suggests that different blood types evolved in response to various dietary and environmental factors. According to this theory, individuals with A-Negative blood type have distinct characteristics and specific dietary requirements that set them apart from other blood types.

The A-Negative Profile:

If you possess A-Negative blood, you share certain genetic traits with other A-Blood Type individuals, which influence your body's response to food and lifestyle choices. Individuals with A-Negative blood type are believed to have ancestors who were primarily agrarian, relying on plant-based diets and engaging in moderate physical activity.

The Nutritional Recommendations for A-Negative:

The Blood Type Diet proposes that A-Negative individuals thrive on a primarily plant-based diet, rich in fresh fruits, vegetables, whole grains, and lean proteins. Emphasizing organic and locally sourced produce is also suggested to optimize nutrient intake and reduce exposure to potentially harmful chemicals.

The Benefits of Following Your Blood Type Diet:

By aligning your food choices with your A-Negative blood type, you may experience a range of potential benefits, including improved digestion, enhanced immune function, increased energy levels, and better overall health. The diet aims to reduce inflammation and promote better weight management, contributing to a sense of well-being and vitality.

Personalizing Your Culinary Journey:

In the following chapters of this part, we will present a selection of customized and delectable recipes designed specifically for A-Negative individuals. These recipes not only cater to your unique nutritional needs but also focus on maximizing taste, texture, and visual appeal.

Cooking with Passion and Purpose:

Remember that the key to success on the Blood Type Diet lies in embracing a balanced and varied approach to your meals. We encourage you to cook with passion and purpose, savoring each bite as you nourish your body and mind.

So, let's embark on this exciting culinary adventure together and discover the joy of eating in harmony with your A-Negative blood type. Get ready to delight in a plethora of delicious and healthful recipes that will make your taste buds sing and your body thank you for the nourishment it deserves. Let's begin!

- Health Benefits and Considerations for Blood Type A-Negative

Understanding the unique characteristics of your A-Negative blood type is essential for making informed choices about your health and well-being. In this section, we will explore the specific health benefits and considerations associated with the Blood Type A-Negative, shedding light on how dietary and lifestyle choices can contribute to a healthier and more vibrant life.

Health Benefits of Blood Type A-Negative:

1. Plant-Based Diet Synergy: A-Negative individuals are believed to have a genetic predisposition for a more plant-based diet. Embracing this dietary approach can lead to numerous health benefits, including improved digestion, increased energy levels, and better weight management.

2. Enhanced Immune Function: Consuming a diet rich in fruits, vegetables, and whole grains can boost your immune system, helping you better fend off infections and illnesses.

3. Reduced Cardiovascular Risk: The Blood Type A-Negative diet focuses on lean proteins, healthy fats, and complex carbohydrates, potentially contributing to improved heart health and reduced risk of cardiovascular diseases.

4. Weight Management: A plant-based diet, coupled with moderate physical activity, may aid in maintaining a healthy weight and reducing the risk of obesity-related conditions.

5. Lowered Inflammation: By avoiding certain foods that may trigger inflammation for A-Negative individuals, the Blood Type Diet may help reduce inflammatory responses in the body.

Considerations for Blood Type A-Negative:

1. Sensitive Digestion: A-Negative individuals may have a more sensitive digestive system, particularly when it comes to handling certain animal proteins and dairy products. Choosing plant-based proteins and dairy alternatives may be beneficial for those with digestive sensitivities.

2. Gluten Sensitivity: Some individuals with A-Negative blood type may experience gluten sensitivity or intolerance. It is advisable to pay attention to how your body responds to gluten-containing foods and consider gluten-free alternatives when necessary.

3. Stress Response: A-Negative individuals may be more prone to stress, and stress management techniques, such as meditation and yoga, can be essential for overall well-being.

4. Regular Physical Activity: Engaging in regular physical activity is highly beneficial for

A-Negative individuals. Consider activities such as walking, yoga, or other forms of moderate exercise to support both physical and mental health.

5. Mindful Eating: Practicing mindful eating, savoring each bite, and listening to your body's cues can help you make healthier food choices and maintain a balanced diet.

Embracing the Blood Type A-Negative Lifestyle:

By recognizing and embracing the unique health benefits and considerations associated with your A-Negative blood type, you have the opportunity to take charge of your well-being. By following the Blood Type A-Negative Diet and making conscious lifestyle choices, you can nourish your body, support your immune system, and promote overall vitality.

As you explore the recipes in this part of the cookbook, keep in mind the health benefits specific to your A-Negative blood type. Enjoy the journey of discovering flavors that align with your genetic heritage, and relish the sense of well-being that comes from making choices that honor your individuality. Remember, the path to optimal health lies in embracing the synergy between your blood type and the food you consume. Let's continue this exciting culinary adventure together!

Chapter 1:

The Basics of Blood Type A-Negative Diet

- What Makes Blood Type A-Negative Unique?

In this chapter, we will explore the distinctive characteristics that make Blood Type A-Negative unique and how understanding these traits can guide your dietary choices for optimal health and well-being.

The A-Negative Blood Type Profile:

Blood Type A-Negative individuals inherit a specific set of genetic markers that differentiate them from other blood types. They belong to the A-Blood Group, characterized by the presence of A antigens on the surface of their red blood cells and the absence of Rh factor (Rh-negative). Let's delve into the key characteristics that set Blood Type A-Negative individuals apart:

1. Agrarian Heritage: The A-Negative blood type is believed to have originated from ancient agrarian societies. Those with this blood type are thought to be descendants of individuals who relied heavily on farming and agricultural practices, consuming diets rich in plant-based foods.

2. Sensitive Digestion: A-Negative individuals tend to have a more sensitive digestive system, which means certain foods may be better tolerated than others. Understanding these nuances can help in making dietary choices that support optimal digestion and overall well-being.

3. Balanced Diet Approach: The Blood Type A-Negative Diet emphasizes a balanced approach to nutrition, focusing on a predominantly plant-based diet with moderate intake of animal proteins. This dietary approach is believed to align better with the genetic heritage of A-Negative individuals.

4. Lower Meat Tolerance: Unlike some other blood types that can thrive on diets with higher meat consumption, A-Negative individuals may find that excessive meat intake can lead to digestive discomfort and potential health issues. Thus, opting for leaner, plant-based protein sources is generally recommended.

5. Mind-Body Connection: A-Negative individuals may have a strong mind-body connection, making stress management and mindful practices essential for maintaining overall health and harmony.

The Benefits of Following the Blood Type A-Negative Diet:

Adhering to the Blood Type A-Negative Diet can offer a range of potential benefits, including:

1. Improved Digestion: By aligning your diet with your A-Negative blood type, you may experience better digestion and reduced digestive discomfort.

2. Enhanced Immune Function: Consuming a diet rich in plant-based foods can boost your immune system, supporting your body's ability to defend against infections and illnesses.

3. Weight Management: The balanced and plant-focused approach of the A-Negative Diet may aid in weight management and overall wellness.

4. Reduced Inflammation: Avoiding foods that may trigger inflammation for A-Negative individuals can contribute to a lower inflammatory response.

5. Increased Energy Levels: A diet aligned with your blood type may provide sustained energy throughout the day, supporting your daily activities and overall vitality.

Understanding Your Blood Type for Optimal Health:

Understanding the unique characteristics of Blood Type A-Negative empowers you to make dietary choices that cater to your specific genetic makeup. By embracing the synergies between your blood type and your diet, you can unlock the potential for improved health and well-being. In the following chapters of this book, we will delve deeper into the foods to emphasize and avoid for A-Negative individuals, providing a wide array of delicious and nutritious recipes tailored to support your health goals. Let's embark on this journey together and embrace the beauty of eating in harmony with our unique blood type!

- Foods to Emphasize for A-Negative Individuals

Foods to Emphasize for A-Negative Individuals
In this chapter, we will explore the foods that are beneficial and supportive for individuals with Blood Type A-Negative. Understanding these foods can help you make informed choices to optimize your health and well-being.

1. Plant-Based Foods:

A-Negative individuals thrive on a predominantly plant-based diet. Emphasize a wide variety of fresh fruits and vegetables in your meals. Aim for a colorful plate that includes leafy greens, broccoli, carrots, bell peppers, berries, and other nutrient-dense produce. These foods are rich in vitamins, minerals, and antioxidants that support your immune system and overall health.

2. Whole Grains:

Incorporate whole grains into your diet, such as quinoa, brown rice, oats, and millet. These grains provide sustained energy and are a great source of fiber, promoting healthy digestion and supporting weight management.

3. Legumes:

Legumes like lentils, chickpeas, and black beans are excellent sources of plant-based protein for A-Negative individuals. They also offer essential minerals like iron and zinc, contributing to overall vitality.

4. Nuts and Seeds:

Include a variety of nuts and seeds in your diet, such as almonds, walnuts, chia seeds, and flaxseeds. These provide healthy fats, protein, and essential nutrients that are beneficial for heart health and brain function.

5. Plant-Based Proteins:

Opt for plant-based protein sources, such as tofu, tempeh, and edamame, which are easier on your sensitive digestive system compared to heavy animal proteins. Incorporate these into stir-fries, salads, or even as a meat alternative in your favorite dishes.

6. Healthy Fats:

Consume healthy fats from sources like avocados, olive oil, and coconut oil. These fats support brain function, aid in nutrient absorption, and promote healthy skin and hair.

7. Herbal Teas:

Herbal teas, such as chamomile, peppermint, and ginger tea, can be soothing and calming for

A-Negative individuals. They can help with stress management and support your sensitive digestive system.

8. Fermented Foods:
Include fermented foods like sauerkraut, kimchi, and miso in your diet. These foods support gut health and enhance digestion by providing beneficial probiotics.

9. Seafood:
For animal protein choices, lean seafood options like salmon, trout, and sardines are better suited for A-Negative individuals. Seafood provides omega-3 fatty acids, which are essential for heart health and brain function.

10. Dairy Alternatives:
If you enjoy dairy, opt for alternatives like almond milk, coconut milk, or oat milk. These dairy-free options are gentler on your digestive system and provide essential nutrients like calcium and vitamin D.

By emphasizing these foods in your daily meals, you can create a well-balanced and nourishing diet that complements your A-Negative blood type. Remember to enjoy a wide variety of flavors and textures, making each meal a delightful and healthful experience. In the next chapter, we will explore the foods to avoid or limit for A-Negative individuals, helping you make informed choices to support your unique nutritional needs. Let's continue this journey toward optimal health and wellness together!

- Foods to Avoid or Limit for A-Negative Individuals

In this section, we will look into some foods that may be less compatible with the A-Negative blood type. Being aware of these foods can help you make mindful choices to support your health and well-being.

1. Red Meat:
A-Negative individuals may find that red meat, such as beef and lamb, is harder to digest and may lead to digestive discomfort. It is advisable

to limit the consumption of red meat or choose leaner cuts if included in your diet.

2. Processed Meats:
Processed meats like bacon, sausages, and deli meats contain additives and preservatives that can be challenging for A-Negative individuals' sensitive digestive systems. It is best to avoid or limit these processed meats.

3. Dairy Products:
Dairy products, especially from cow's milk, can be less compatible with A-Negative individuals. These may contribute to digestive issues and inflammation. Consider dairy alternatives like almond milk or coconut milk.

4. Wheat-Based Products:
A-Negative individuals may have a higher sensitivity to gluten found in wheat-based products like bread, pasta, and baked goods. Consider gluten-free alternatives like quinoa, rice, or gluten-free grains.

5. Corn and Corn Products:

Corn and corn-based products may not be as well-tolerated by A-Negative individuals. Opt for other grains and vegetables instead.

6. Nightshade Vegetables:
Some A-Negative individuals may experience sensitivity to nightshade vegetables like tomatoes, potatoes, and eggplants. Observe how your body responds to these vegetables and consider alternatives if needed.

7. Certain Beans and Legumes:
While legumes, in general, are beneficial, A-Negative individuals may find certain beans, such as kidney beans, to be less compatible with their digestion. Focus on other legumes that suit your system better.

8. Oranges and Orange Juice:
Oranges and orange juice can be acidic and may not be ideal for A-Negative individuals, especially if you experience acid reflux or heartburn. Opt for other vitamin C-rich fruits like berries or kiwis.

9. Bananas:

While bananas are a favorite fruit for many, some A-Negative individuals may experience bloating or digestive discomfort after consuming them. If you notice this, consider reducing your banana intake.

10. Excessive Salt and Processed Foods:
High-sodium and processed foods may contribute to water retention and elevated blood pressure for A-Negative individuals. Choose whole, unprocessed foods whenever possible.

11. Sugary Treats:
Excessive sugary treats can lead to fluctuations in energy levels and may not support the overall well-being of A-Negative individuals. Enjoy sweets in moderation and opt for healthier alternatives like fruit-based desserts.

By being mindful of these foods and making informed choices, you can create a diet that aligns with your A-Negative blood type, supporting your unique nutritional needs and promoting optimal health. In the following chapters, we will explore a wide array of delicious and nutritious recipes tailored specifically for A-Negative individuals, making your culinary journey both enjoyable and healthful. Let's continue this exciting adventure toward better health and vitality together!

Chapter 2:

Breakfast Delights

- Berry and Almond Milk Smoothie

Start your day with a burst of deliciousness and nourishment with our Berry and Almond Milk Smoothie—a refreshing and nutrient-packed breakfast option tailored for A-Negative individuals. This smoothie is not only delightful to the taste buds but also provides a perfect balance of plant-based goodness to kick-start your morning.

Health Tip: The Healthy Components of the Major Ingredients

Before we dive into the recipe, let's explore the healthy components of the major ingredients in this Berry and Almond Milk Smoothie, showcasing how each element contributes to your well-being:

Berries: Whether it's strawberries, blueberries, raspberries, or blackberries, these colorful fruits are rich in antioxidants, vitamins, and fiber. They help combat oxidative stress, support immune function, and promote a healthy gut.

Almond Milk: Made from almonds, almond milk is a fantastic dairy-free alternative that provides essential nutrients like vitamin E, calcium, and healthy fats. It is gentle on the digestive system and complements the A-Negative dietary profile.

Banana: Despite being limited for some A-Negative individuals, bananas in moderation offer potassium, vitamin B6, and natural sweetness. They also lend a creamy texture to the smoothie.

Chia Seeds: These tiny powerhouses pack omega-3 fatty acids, fiber, and protein. They promote satiety, support heart health, and help stabilize blood sugar levels.

Greek Yogurt (Optional): If you tolerate dairy well, adding a dollop of Greek yogurt can provide probiotics and protein, supporting gut health and overall digestion.

Ingredients:
- 1 cup mixed berries (strawberries, blueberries, or any favorites)
- 1 ripe banana (use in moderation if well-tolerated)
- 1 tablespoon chia seeds
- 1 cup unsweetened almond milk
- 1/4 cup Greek yogurt (optional, if tolerated)
- Ice cubes (optional, for a chilled smoothie)

Instructions:

1. In a blender, add the mixed berries, peeled banana (if using), chia seeds, almond milk, and Greek yogurt (if using).

2. If you prefer a chilled smoothie, you can also add a few ice cubes to the blender.

3. Blend all the ingredients until smooth and creamy, ensuring that the berries and chia seeds are fully incorporated.

4. Take a moment to appreciate the vibrant color and enticing aroma of your Berry and Almond Milk Smoothie.

5. Pour the smoothie into a tall glass and, if you like, garnish it with a few fresh berries or a sprinkle of chia seeds.

6. Sip and savor the refreshing goodness of your Berry and Almond Milk Smoothie, enjoying the delicate balance of sweet and tangy flavors.

7. Embrace this nutritious and energizing breakfast, knowing that you are nourishing your body with wholesome ingredients that align with your A-Negative blood type.

Note: Feel free to customize your smoothie based on personal preferences or ingredient availability. You can add a drizzle of honey for added sweetness or throw in a handful of spinach for an extra nutrient boost.

This Berry and Almond Milk Smoothie is the perfect way to start your day, providing you with a wealth of nutrients and setting a positive tone for the hours ahead. Let's explore more delightful breakfast options and continue our culinary journey to embrace the synergy between your blood type and the foods you consume. Enjoy!

- Sweet Potato Hash with Poached Eggs

Indulge in a hearty and satisfying breakfast with our Sweet Potato Hash with Poached Eggs—an A-Negative-friendly dish that combines the goodness of sweet potatoes, colorful vegetables, and perfectly poached eggs. This nutrient-rich breakfast will keep you fueled and energized throughout the morning.

Health Tip: The Healthy Components of the Major Ingredients

Let's explore the healthy components of the major ingredients in this Sweet Potato Hash with Poached Eggs, highlighting how each element contributes to your well-being:

Sweet Potatoes: Packed with vitamins, minerals, and fiber, sweet potatoes are a fantastic source of complex carbohydrates. They provide sustained energy, support digestive health, and contain antioxidants to boost your immune system.

Colorful Vegetables: Bell peppers, onions, and spinach add a vibrant array of nutrients to the dish. These vegetables supply vitamins, minerals, and phytonutrients, promoting overall health and vitality.

Eggs: Poached eggs provide high-quality protein, essential amino acids, and healthy fats. They also offer essential nutrients like vitamin B12, choline, and selenium, supporting brain function and cellular health.

Ingredients:
- 2 medium sweet potatoes, peeled and diced
- 1 red bell pepper, diced
- 1 yellow bell pepper, diced
- 1 small red onion, thinly sliced
- 2 cups fresh baby spinach
- 2 tablespoons olive oil
- Salt and pepper to taste
- 4 large eggs
- Fresh parsley or cilantro for garnish (optional)

Instructions:

1. In a large skillet, heat 1 tablespoon of olive oil over medium heat.

2. Add the diced sweet potatoes to the skillet, and season with salt and pepper. Cook until the sweet potatoes are tender and lightly browned, about 10-12 minutes.

3. Push the sweet potatoes to one side of the skillet, and add the remaining 1 tablespoon of olive oil to the other side.

4. Toss in the diced red and yellow bell peppers and sliced red onion. Saute until the vegetables are softened and slightly caramelized, about 5-7 minutes.

5. Stir in the fresh baby spinach, and cook until it wilts down and combines with the rest of the hash.

6. In a separate saucepan, bring water to a gentle simmer. Add a splash of vinegar to the water (optional) to help the eggs coagulate better during poaching.

7. Crack each egg into a small bowl. Create a gentle whirlpool in the simmering water using a spoon, and carefully slide each egg into the center of the whirlpool. Poach the eggs for about 3-4 minutes for a soft, runny yolk or longer for a firmer yolk.

8. Using a slotted spoon, carefully remove the poached eggs from the water and place them on a plate lined with a paper towel to drain any excess water.

9. Plate the Sweet Potato Hash, and top each serving with a perfectly poached egg.

10. Garnish with fresh parsley or cilantro, if desired, and add a sprinkle of salt and pepper to taste.

11. Admire the beautiful colors and enticing aroma of your Sweet Potato Hash with Poached Eggs.

12. Dig into this wholesome and flavorsome breakfast, savoring the delightful combination of sweet potatoes, colorful vegetables, and the richness of the poached eggs.

Note: You can also get creative with this dish by adding your favorite herbs or spices for added flavor. Feel free to experiment with different vegetables to suit your preferences or seasonal produce availability.

Enjoy the satisfying and nutritious Sweet Potato Hash with Poached Eggs, knowing that you have started your day with a delicious and healthful meal that supports your A-Negative blood type. Let's continue our culinary exploration and embrace the goodness of foods that resonate with your unique genetic heritage!

- Greek Yogurt Parfait with Honey and Nuts

Indulge in a delightful and protein-packed breakfast with our Greek Yogurt Parfait with Honey and Nuts—a delectable A-Negative-friendly dish that combines the creaminess of Greek yogurt with the natural sweetness of honey and the crunch of nutritious nuts. This parfait is a perfect balance of flavors and textures to start your day on a delicious note.

Health Tip: The Healthy Components of the Major Ingredients

Let's explore the healthy components of the major ingredients in this Greek Yogurt Parfait with Honey and Nuts, highlighting how each element contributes to your well-being:

Greek Yogurt: Greek yogurt is a nutritional powerhouse, providing protein, calcium, probiotics, and vitamin B12. It supports gut health, strengthens bones, and aids in digestion.

Honey: As a natural sweetener, honey offers a touch of sweetness without refined sugars. It also contains antioxidants and may provide soothing properties for the throat and respiratory system.

Nuts: Almonds, walnuts, or any preferred nuts in the parfait supply healthy fats, protein, and essential nutrients like vitamin E and magnesium. They promote heart health, brain function, and overall well-being.

Ingredients:
- 1 cup Greek yogurt (plain or vanilla-flavored)
- 2 tablespoons honey (adjust to taste)
- 1/4 cup mixed nuts (almonds, walnuts, or any favorites), chopped
- 1/2 cup fresh berries (blueberries, strawberries, or raspberries)

- 1 tablespoon chia seeds (optional, for added texture)
- A dash of cinnamon (optional, for extra flavor)

Instructions:

1. In a small bowl, mix the Greek yogurt with honey until well combined. Adjust the amount of honey to suit your desired level of sweetness.

2. If you choose to add chia seeds, stir them into the Greek yogurt and let the mixture sit for a few minutes to allow the chia seeds to absorb some liquid and create a pudding-like texture.

3. In a separate pan, lightly toast the chopped nuts over medium heat until they become fragrant and slightly golden. This step enhances the nutty flavor and adds crunch to the parfait.

4. Layer the Greek yogurt mixture in a glass or a bowl, alternating with fresh berries and toasted nuts.

5. Repeat the layering process until all the ingredients are used, creating beautiful layers of creamy yogurt, sweet berries, and crunchy nuts.

6. Sprinkle a dash of cinnamon on top if desired, for an extra touch of warmth and flavor.

7. Take a moment to admire the vibrant colors and inviting layers of your Greek Yogurt Parfait with Honey and Nuts.

8. Grab a spoon and savor the delightful medley of textures and tastes in every spoonful.

Note: Feel free to customize your parfait with other favorite toppings like granola, shredded coconut, or even a drizzle of dark chocolate for an indulgent treat.

Enjoy the wholesome and scrumptious Greek Yogurt Parfait with Honey and Nuts, knowing that you've embraced a breakfast that nourishes your body and aligns with your A-Negative blood type. Let's continue to explore a variety of delightful breakfast options and savor the goodness of foods that resonate with your unique genetic heritage!

- Buckwheat Pancakes with Fresh Fruit

Treat yourself to a stack of fluffy and nutritious Buckwheat Pancakes with Fresh Fruit—a mouthwatering A-Negative-friendly breakfast that combines the goodness of buckwheat flour with the natural sweetness of fresh fruit. These pancakes are not only delicious but also packed with essential nutrients to fuel your morning.

Health Tip: The Healthy Components of the Major Ingredients

Let's explore the healthy components of the major ingredients in these Buckwheat Pancakes with Fresh Fruit, showcasing how each element contributes to your well-being:

Buckwheat Flour: Buckwheat is a pseudo-grain that is gluten-free and rich in fiber, vitamins, and minerals. It provides sustained energy, supports heart health, and aids in digestion.

Fresh Fruit: Whether it's sliced bananas, blueberries, or any seasonal fruit, fresh fruit adds natural sweetness, vitamins, antioxidants, and fiber to the pancakes.

Ingredients:
- 1 cup buckwheat flour
- 2 tablespoons coconut sugar (or preferred sweetener)
- 1 teaspoon baking powder
- 1/2 teaspoon baking soda
- 1/4 teaspoon salt
- 1 cup almond milk (or any preferred milk)
- 1 large egg (or flax egg for a vegan option)
- 2 tablespoons melted coconut oil (or any preferred oil)
- Fresh fruit of your choice for topping (blueberries, strawberries, bananas, etc.)
- Maple syrup or honey for drizzling

Instructions:

1. In a large mixing bowl, whisk together the buckwheat flour, coconut sugar, baking powder, baking soda, and salt.

2. In a separate bowl, whisk the almond milk, egg (or flax egg), and melted coconut oil.

3. Pour the wet ingredients into the dry ingredients, and gently stir until just combined. Be careful not to overmix; some lumps are okay.

4. Let the batter sit for a few minutes to allow the buckwheat flour to hydrate.

5. Heat a non-stick skillet or griddle over medium heat. Lightly grease the surface with coconut oil or cooking spray.

6. Pour about 1/4 cup of the pancake batter onto the hot skillet for each pancake.

7. Cook until bubbles form on the surface of the pancake and the edges look set, about 2-3 minutes.

8. Flip the pancakes and cook the other side until golden brown, about 1-2 minutes more.

9. Stack the cooked pancakes on a plate, and keep them warm in a low oven until all the batter is used.

10. Top the Buckwheat Pancakes with an assortment of fresh fruit, such as blueberries, strawberries, or banana slices.

11. Drizzle your preferred amount of maple syrup or honey over the pancakes for added sweetness.

12. Admire the beautiful presentation and delightful aroma of your Buckwheat Pancakes with Fresh Fruit.

13. Take your first bite and enjoy the fluffy texture, nutty flavor, and burst of fruity goodness in every mouthful.

Note: These pancakes are versatile, so feel free to customize them with additional toppings like a dollop of Greek yogurt, a sprinkle of chia seeds, or a dusting of cinnamon for added flavor.

Indulge in the wholesome and delightful Buckwheat Pancakes with Fresh Fruit, knowing that you've started your day with a breakfast that aligns with your A-Negative blood type and provides you with essential nutrients. Let's continue our culinary journey and explore more delectable breakfast options to support your overall health and well-being!

Chapter 3:

Scrumptious Lunches

- Lentil and Spinach Salad

Delight in a nourishing and flavorful Lentil and Spinach Salad—a satisfying A-Negative-friendly lunch that combines protein-packed lentils with vibrant spinach and a zesty dressing. This wholesome salad is not only a feast for the taste buds but also a source of essential nutrients to keep you energized throughout the day.

Health Tip: The Healthy Components of the Major Ingredients

Let's explore the healthy components of the major ingredients in this Lentil and Spinach Salad, showcasing how each element contributes to your well-being:

Lentils: Lentils are a fantastic plant-based source of protein, fiber, iron, and folate. They support digestive health, stabilize blood sugar levels, and provide lasting energy.

Spinach: Spinach is a leafy green rich in vitamins A, C, and K, as well as iron and antioxidants. It supports bone health, boosts immunity, and promotes healthy skin.

Ingredients:
- 1 cup cooked green or brown lentils
- 2 cups fresh baby spinach leaves
- 1/2 cup cherry tomatoes, halved
- 1/4 cup diced cucumber
- 1/4 cup thinly sliced red onion
- 2 tablespoons crumbled feta cheese (optional, if tolerated)
- 2 tablespoons chopped fresh parsley or cilantro
- 2 tablespoons extra-virgin olive oil
- 1 tablespoon fresh lemon juice
- 1 teaspoon Dijon mustard
- 1 clove garlic, minced
- Salt and pepper to taste

Instructions:

1. In a large mixing bowl, combine the cooked lentils, fresh baby spinach, cherry tomatoes, diced cucumber, sliced red onion, and crumbled feta cheese (if using).

2. In a small jar with a lid, prepare the dressing by combining the extra-virgin olive oil, fresh lemon juice, Dijon mustard, minced garlic, salt, and pepper. Secure the lid and shake the jar vigorously to emulsify the dressing.

3. Drizzle the dressing over the lentil and spinach mixture, and gently toss until all the ingredients are coated with the zesty dressing.

4. Add the chopped fresh parsley or cilantro to the salad and toss again to incorporate the herb's fresh flavor.

5. Taste the salad and adjust the seasoning, adding more salt or pepper if needed.

6. Let the flavors meld together for a few minutes, allowing the dressing to infuse the salad with its delightful taste.

7. Transfer the Lentil and Spinach Salad to a serving dish or individual plates, creating an appetizing presentation.

8. Take a moment to admire the vibrant colors and nutrient-packed ingredients in your Lentil and Spinach Salad.

9. Dig into this wholesome and flavorful salad, relishing the earthy lentils, refreshing spinach, and the tangy notes of the zesty dressing.

Note: Feel free to customize this salad with other preferred vegetables or add nuts or seeds for added texture and nutrition.

Savor the delightful and nutrient-rich Lentil and Spinach Salad, knowing that you've chosen a lunch that aligns with your A-Negative blood type and provides you with essential nutrients. Let's continue our culinary exploration and discover more scrumptious lunch options to support your overall health and well-being!

- Vegetable and Quinoa Stuffed Peppers

Enjoy a delectable and nutritious lunch with our Vegetable and Quinoa Stuffed Peppers—a delightful A-Negative-friendly dish that combines colorful vegetables and protein-rich quinoa in a deliciously wholesome package. These stuffed peppers are not only visually appealing but also packed with essential nutrients to keep you satisfied and energized.

Health Tip: The Healthy Components of the Major Ingredients

Let's explore the healthy components of the major ingredients in these Vegetable and Quinoa Stuffed Peppers, showcasing how each element contributes to your well-being:

Bell Peppers: Colorful bell peppers are rich in vitamins A and C, antioxidants, and fiber. They support eye health, boost immunity, and aid in digestion.

Quinoa: Quinoa is a complete protein that provides all nine essential amino acids. It is also a good source of fiber, iron, and magnesium, supporting muscle health and energy production.

Ingredients:
- 4 large bell peppers (red, yellow, or orange)
- 1 cup cooked quinoa
- 1 cup diced zucchini
- 1 cup diced eggplant
- 1 cup diced tomatoes
- 1/2 cup diced red onion
- 2 cloves garlic, minced
- 2 tablespoons chopped fresh basil or parsley
- 2 tablespoons extra-virgin olive oil
- 1/4 teaspoon dried oregano
- Salt and pepper to taste
- 1/2 cup crumbled feta cheese (optional, if tolerated)

Instructions:

1. Preheat your oven to 375°F (190°C).

2. Cut the tops off the bell peppers, and remove the seeds and membranes from the inside.

3. In a large skillet, heat one tablespoon of olive oil over medium heat.

4. Add the diced zucchini, eggplant, tomatoes, red onion, and minced garlic to the skillet. Season with dried oregano, salt, and pepper.

5. Sauté the vegetables until they are tender and lightly browned, about 8-10 minutes.

6. In a separate bowl, combine the cooked quinoa with the sautéed vegetables and chopped fresh basil or parsley. Mix well to incorporate all the flavors.

7. If you choose to add feta cheese, gently fold in the crumbled feta into the quinoa and vegetable mixture.

8. Stuff each bell pepper with the quinoa and vegetable mixture, packing it tightly.

9. Place the stuffed peppers in a baking dish, and drizzle the remaining olive oil over the tops.

10. Cover the baking dish with aluminum foil, and bake the stuffed peppers in the preheated oven for 25-30 minutes, or until the peppers are tender.

11. Remove the foil during the last 5 minutes of baking to allow the tops to brown slightly.

12. Take the stuffed peppers out of the oven, and let them cool for a few minutes.

13. Plate the Vegetable and Quinoa Stuffed Peppers, and garnish with additional fresh herbs if desired.

14. Admire the vibrant colors and enticing aroma of your Vegetable and Quinoa Stuffed Peppers.

15. Cut into each pepper, and savor the delightful combination of flavorful vegetables, protein-packed quinoa, and the potential creaminess of feta cheese.

Note: Feel free to experiment with different vegetables or spices to suit your taste preferences or seasonal produce availability.

Enjoy the delicious and nutrient-dense Vegetable and Quinoa Stuffed Peppers, knowing that you've chosen a lunch that aligns with your A-Negative blood type and provides you with essential nutrients for a nourishing meal. Let's continue our culinary journey and explore more scrumptious lunch options to support your overall health and well-being!

- Grilled Chicken Salad with Mixed Greens

Savor the flavors of a refreshing and protein-packed Grilled Chicken Salad with Mixed Greens—a delightful A-Negative-friendly lunch that combines tender grilled chicken with a medley of crisp mixed greens and a tantalizing dressing. This wholesome salad is a perfect balance of textures and tastes to keep you feeling light and energized.

Health Tip: The Healthy Components of the Major Ingredients

Let's explore the healthy components of the major ingredients in this Grilled Chicken Salad with Mixed Greens, highlighting how each element contributes to your well-being:

Grilled Chicken: Lean grilled chicken breast is an excellent source of high-quality protein, essential amino acids, and vitamin B6. It supports muscle health, promotes satiety, and aids in tissue repair.

Mixed Greens: A combination of fresh baby spinach, arugula, and lettuces provides an array of vitamins, minerals, and antioxidants. These leafy greens support digestion, hydrate the body, and nourish the skin.

Ingredients:
- 2 boneless, skinless chicken breasts
- 4 cups mixed greens (baby spinach, arugula, lettuce, etc.)
- 1 cup cherry tomatoes, halved
- 1/2 cucumber, sliced
- 1/4 red onion, thinly sliced
- 1/4 cup crumbled goat cheese or feta cheese (optional, if tolerated)
- 2 tablespoons sliced almonds or any preferred nuts (toasted, if desired)
- 2 tablespoons extra-virgin olive oil
- 2 tablespoons balsamic vinegar
- 1 teaspoon Dijon mustard
- 1 clove garlic, minced
- Salt and pepper to taste

Instructions:

1. Preheat your grill or grill pan to medium-high heat.

2. Season the chicken breasts with salt and pepper, and grill them until they are cooked through and have beautiful grill marks, about 4-5 minutes per side.

3. Remove the grilled chicken from the heat, and let it rest for a few minutes before slicing it into thin strips.

4. In a large salad bowl, combine the mixed greens, cherry tomatoes, cucumber, and thinly sliced red onion.

5. In a small jar with a lid, prepare the dressing by combining the extra-virgin olive oil, balsamic vinegar, Dijon mustard, minced garlic, salt, and pepper. Secure the lid and shake the jar vigorously to emulsify the dressing.

6. Drizzle the dressing over the salad, and toss gently to ensure all the ingredients are coated with the flavorful dressing.

7. If you choose to add cheese, sprinkle the crumbled goat cheese or feta cheese over the salad.

8. Top the Grilled Chicken Salad with the sliced grilled chicken, adding a generous handful of

sliced almonds or preferred nuts for added crunch and texture.

9. Take a moment to admire the colorful arrangement and tantalizing aroma of your Grilled Chicken Salad with Mixed Greens.

10. Serve the salad immediately, allowing everyone to enjoy the fresh and crisp goodness of the ingredients.

Note: You can customize your salad with additional vegetables or fruits for extra flavor and nutrition. Grilled asparagus, avocado slices, or dried cranberries are excellent choices.

Relish the delightful and nutrient-rich Grilled Chicken Salad with Mixed Greens, knowing that you've chosen a lunch that aligns with your A-Negative blood type and provides you with essential nutrients. Let's continue our culinary exploration and discover more scrumptious lunch options to support your overall health and well-being!

- Miso Soup with Tofu and Seaweed

Warm your soul and nourish your body with a comforting bowl of Miso Soup with Tofu and Seaweed—a delightful A-Negative-friendly lunch that combines the umami goodness of miso with silky tofu and nutrient-rich seaweed. This soothing soup is not only delicious but also a source of essential minerals and vitamins to keep you feeling revitalized.

Health Tip: The Healthy Components of the Major Ingredients

Let's explore the healthy components of the major ingredients in this Miso Soup with Tofu and Seaweed, showcasing how each element contributes to your well-being:

Miso Paste: Miso is a fermented soybean paste that offers probiotics, protein, and antioxidants. It supports gut health, aids in digestion, and provides a savory flavor base for the soup.

Tofu: Silken tofu is a versatile plant-based protein that is rich in calcium and iron. It supports bone health, muscle function, and overall well-being.

Seaweed: Seaweed, such as wakame or nori, is abundant in vitamins A, C, and K, as well as iodine and other minerals. It promotes thyroid health, boosts immunity, and provides a hint of oceanic flavor.

Ingredients:
- 4 cups vegetable or mushroom broth (or any preferred broth)
- 3 tablespoons miso paste (white or red miso, to taste)
- 1 cup cubed silken tofu
- 1/4 cup dried wakame seaweed (or any preferred seaweed)
- 2 green onions, thinly sliced
- 1 tablespoon soy sauce (optional, for added depth of flavor)
- 1 tablespoon sesame oil
- 1 teaspoon grated fresh ginger
- 1 clove garlic, minced

- A pinch of red pepper flakes (optional, for a hint of heat)
- Freshly ground black pepper to taste

Instructions:

1. In a medium-sized pot, bring the vegetable or mushroom broth to a gentle simmer over medium heat.

2. In a small bowl, dilute the miso paste with a ladleful of the warm broth to create a smooth paste.

3. Gradually whisk the diluted miso paste into the simmering broth until it dissolves completely.

4. Add the cubed silken tofu and dried wakame seaweed to the soup. Let them simmer gently for a few minutes to rehydrate the seaweed and warm the tofu.

5. Stir in the thinly sliced green onions, grated fresh ginger, minced garlic, and a pinch of red pepper flakes (if using). These aromatic

additions infuse the soup with a delightful depth of flavor.

6. If you prefer a slightly richer taste, add soy sauce to the soup, adjusting the amount to your liking.

7. Drizzle sesame oil over the soup, adding a hint of nuttiness to the broth.

8. Season the Miso Soup with freshly ground black pepper to taste.

9. Ladle the warm Miso Soup with Tofu and Seaweed into serving bowls, and enjoy its comforting aroma.

10. Sip the soothing and nutritious broth, relishing the umami taste of the miso, the velvety texture of tofu, and the oceanic essence of seaweed.

Note: Feel free to customize your soup with additional vegetables like sliced mushrooms, baby spinach, or julienned carrots for added nutrition and color.

Relish the comforting and nutrient-rich Miso Soup with Tofu and Seaweed, knowing that you've chosen a lunch that aligns with your A-Negative blood type and provides you with essential nutrients for a nourishing meal. Let's continue our culinary journey and explore more scrumptious lunch options to support your overall health and well-being!

Chapter 4:

Delectable Dinners

- Baked Cod with Herbed Quinoa

Indulge in a delectable and healthful dinner with our Baked Cod with Herbed Quinoa—a mouthwatering A-Negative-friendly dish that combines tender baked cod with flavorful quinoa infused with fragrant herbs. This dinner is not only a feast for the taste buds but also a source of essential nutrients to support your well-being.

Health Tip: The Healthy Components of the Major Ingredients

Let's explore the healthy components of the major ingredients in this Baked Cod with Herbed Quinoa, showcasing how each element contributes to your well-being:

Cod: Cod is a lean white fish that provides high-quality protein, omega-3 fatty acids, and essential vitamins. It supports heart health, brain function, and overall vitality.

Quinoa: Quinoa is a versatile ancient grain that offers complete protein, dietary fiber, and various minerals. It supports digestive health, stabilizes blood sugar levels, and provides sustained energy.

Ingredients:
- 4 cod fillets (about 4-6 ounces each)
- 1 cup quinoa, rinsed and drained
- 2 cups vegetable or chicken broth (or water)
- 1 tablespoon chopped fresh dill
- 1 tablespoon chopped fresh parsley
- 1 tablespoon chopped fresh chives
- 1 tablespoon lemon juice
- 1 tablespoon extra-virgin olive oil
- 2 cloves garlic, minced
- Salt and pepper to taste
- Lemon wedges for serving

Instructions:

1. Preheat your oven to 375°F (190°C). Line a baking sheet with parchment paper or lightly grease it to prevent sticking.

2. Place the cod fillets on the prepared baking sheet, and drizzle them with half of the lemon juice and extra-virgin olive oil. Season with salt and pepper to taste.

3. Bake the cod in the preheated oven for about 15-20 minutes, or until the fish is opaque and easily flakes with a fork.

4. Remove the baked cod from the oven, and sprinkle the remaining lemon juice over the fillets for a burst of citrusy freshness.

For the Herbed Quinoa:

1. In a medium saucepan, bring the vegetable or chicken broth (or water) to a boil.

2. Add the rinsed quinoa to the boiling broth, and reduce the heat to low.

3. Cover the saucepan with a lid, and let the quinoa simmer for 15-20 minutes, or until the liquid is absorbed and the quinoa is fluffy.

4. Once the quinoa is cooked, fluff it with a fork and stir in the chopped fresh dill, parsley, chives, minced garlic, extra-virgin olive oil, and a sprinkle of salt and pepper.

5. Taste the herbed quinoa and adjust the seasoning or add more fresh herbs to your liking.

To Serve:

1. Plate the Baked Cod with a generous serving of the Herbed Quinoa.

2. Garnish with additional fresh herbs for an appealing presentation.

3. Serve with lemon wedges on the side for squeezing over the cod, enhancing its taste with zesty brightness.

Note: You can customize the herbed quinoa by adding other preferred herbs like basil, cilantro, or thyme for added flavor complexity.

Enjoy the delectable and nutrient-rich Baked Cod with Herbed Quinoa, knowing that you've chosen a dinner that aligns with your A-Negative blood type and provides you with essential nutrients for a satisfying meal. Let's continue our culinary exploration and discover more delightful dinner options to support your overall health and well-being!

- Roasted Vegetable Stir-Fry with Cashews

Embark on a delightful culinary journey with our Roasted Vegetable Stir-Fry with Cashews—a tantalizing A-Negative-friendly dinner that brings together an array of roasted vegetables and crunchy cashews in a flavorful stir-fry. This dinner not only delights the palate but also provides a wealth of essential nutrients for a nourishing meal.

Health Tip: The Healthy Components of the Major Ingredients

Let's explore the healthy components of the major ingredients in this Roasted Vegetable Stir-Fry with Cashews, showcasing how each element contributes to your well-being:

Roasted Vegetables: A medley of colorful vegetables like bell peppers, broccoli, carrots, and zucchini provides an abundance of vitamins, minerals, and antioxidants. They promote eye health, support the immune system, and aid in digestion.

Cashews: Cashews offer heart-healthy monounsaturated fats, protein, and essential minerals like magnesium and zinc. They support brain function, reduce inflammation, and contribute to overall well-being.

Ingredients:
- 2 cups mixed vegetables (bell peppers, broccoli, carrots, zucchini, etc.), chopped
- 1 cup snap peas or snow peas

- 1/2 cup sliced mushrooms
- 1/4 cup sliced red onion
- 1/2 cup raw cashews
- 3 tablespoons low-sodium soy sauce or tamari (for a gluten-free option)
- 1 tablespoon rice vinegar
- 1 tablespoon toasted sesame oil
- 1 tablespoon grated fresh ginger
- 2 cloves garlic, minced
- 1 tablespoon honey or maple syrup (optional, for a touch of sweetness)
- 1 tablespoon cornstarch or arrowroot powder (to thicken the sauce)
- 2 tablespoons sesame seeds (optional, for garnish)
- 2 tablespoons chopped green onions (optional, for garnish)
- Cooked quinoa, brown rice, or noodles for serving

Instructions:

1. Preheat your oven to 400°F (200°C). Line a baking sheet with parchment paper.

2. In a large bowl, toss the chopped mixed vegetables, snap peas, sliced mushrooms, and red onion with 1 tablespoon of toasted sesame oil.

3. Spread the vegetables evenly on the prepared baking sheet, and roast them in the preheated oven for about 15-20 minutes or until they are tender and slightly caramelized.

4. While the vegetables roast, prepare the stir-fry sauce. In a small bowl, whisk together the low-sodium soy sauce or tamari, rice vinegar, grated fresh ginger, minced garlic, and honey or maple syrup (if using).

5. In a separate bowl, mix the cornstarch or arrowroot powder with a tablespoon of water to create a slurry. This will help thicken the sauce.

6. In a large skillet or wok, heat the remaining tablespoon of toasted sesame oil over medium heat.

7. Add the roasted vegetables to the skillet, along with the raw cashews. Stir-fry for a minute or two to combine the flavors.

8. Pour the stir-fry sauce over the vegetables and cashews, and toss everything together until the sauce coats the vegetables evenly.

9. Add the cornstarch or arrowroot slurry to the skillet, and continue to stir-fry for another minute until the sauce thickens and becomes glossy.

10. Sprinkle sesame seeds over the stir-fry for a delightful nutty crunch (if using).

11. Remove the skillet from the heat, and garnish the Roasted Vegetable Stir-Fry with chopped green onions for a pop of color (if using).

12. Serve the flavorful stir-fry over cooked quinoa, brown rice, or noodles for a complete and satisfying meal.

Note: Feel free to customize your stir-fry with other preferred vegetables and adjust the sauce to your taste preferences.

Enjoy the scrumptious and nutrient-rich Roasted Vegetable Stir-Fry with Cashews, knowing that you've chosen a dinner that aligns with your A-Negative blood type and provides you with essential nutrients for a satisfying meal. Let's continue our culinary exploration and discover more delightful dinner options to support your overall health and well-being!

- Portobello Mushroom Marsala

Savor the rich and savory flavors of Portobello Mushroom Marsala—a delightful A-Negative-friendly dinner that elevates meaty Portobello mushrooms in a luscious Marsala wine sauce. This dish not only satisfies your taste buds but also provides a wealth of essential nutrients for a satisfying and comforting meal.

Health Tip: The Healthy Components of the Major Ingredients

Let's explore the healthy components of the major ingredients in this Portobello Mushroom Marsala, showcasing how each element contributes to your well-being:

Portobello Mushrooms: Portobello mushrooms are a low-calorie and nutrient-dense alternative to meat. They provide fiber, vitamins, and minerals, supporting digestive health and overall well-being.

Marsala Wine: Marsala wine lends a rich and complex flavor to the dish. Moderate consumption of wine in cooking has been associated with certain health benefits, including heart health.

Ingredients:
- 4 large Portobello mushrooms, stems removed
- 2 tablespoons olive oil

- 1/4 cup all-purpose flour (or gluten-free flour for a gluten-free option)
- 1 cup vegetable broth
- 1/2 cup Marsala wine
- 1/2 cup sliced cremini mushrooms
- 1/4 cup sliced shallots or onions
- 2 cloves garlic, minced
- 1/4 cup unsweetened almond milk or any preferred milk
- 2 tablespoons chopped fresh parsley
- Salt and pepper to taste
- Cooked quinoa, brown rice, or mashed potatoes for serving

Instructions:

1. Preheat your oven to 375°F (190°C).

2. Place the Portobello mushrooms on a baking sheet, and drizzle them with olive oil. Season with salt and pepper to taste.

3. Bake the Portobello mushrooms in the preheated oven for about 15-20 minutes or until they are tender and slightly caramelized.

4. While the mushrooms bake, prepare the Marsala sauce. In a medium saucepan over medium heat, whisk the flour with the vegetable broth until there are no lumps.

5. Add the Marsala wine to the saucepan, and stir until the mixture is smooth and well combined.

6. Stir in the sliced cremini mushrooms, shallots or onions, and minced garlic.

7. Let the sauce simmer for about 5-7 minutes, or until it thickens slightly and the flavors meld together.

8. Reduce the heat to low, and stir in the unsweetened almond milk or any preferred milk to create a creamy consistency.

9. Add chopped fresh parsley to the Marsala sauce, and season with salt and pepper to taste.

10. Once the Portobello mushrooms are done baking, transfer them to a serving plate.

11. Pour the Marsala sauce over the baked Portobello mushrooms, generously coating them in the rich and flavorful sauce.

12. Serve the Portobello Mushroom Marsala over cooked quinoa, brown rice, or creamy mashed potatoes for a satisfying and well-rounded meal.

Note: Feel free to customize your Portobello Mushroom Marsala with additional herbs or vegetables for added flavor and nutrition.

Indulge in the delectable and nutrient-rich Portobello Mushroom Marsala, knowing that you've chosen a dinner that aligns with your A-Negative blood type and provides you with essential nutrients for a satisfying meal. Let's continue our culinary exploration and discover more delightful dinner options to support your overall health and well-being!

- Tofu and Vegetable Curry

Embark on a flavorful journey with our Tofu and Vegetable Curry—a delightful A-Negative-friendly dinner that brings together the creaminess of tofu and a vibrant array of vegetables in a fragrant curry sauce. This dish not only tantalizes the taste buds but also provides a wealth of essential nutrients for a nourishing and satisfying meal.

Health Tip: The Healthy Components of the Major Ingredients

Let's explore the healthy components of the major ingredients in this Tofu and Vegetable Curry, showcasing how each element contributes to your well-being:

Tofu: Tofu is a versatile plant-based protein made from soybeans. It is a good source of calcium, iron, and amino acids, supporting bone health, energy production, and muscle function.

Vegetables: An assortment of vegetables such as bell peppers, carrots, cauliflower, and peas provides an abundance of vitamins, minerals, and antioxidants. They promote overall health, aid in digestion, and boost immunity.

Curry Spices: The aromatic blend of curry spices, including turmeric, cumin, coriander, and ginger, offers anti-inflammatory properties and adds depth of flavor to the dish.

Ingredients:
- 1 block (14 oz) firm tofu, cubed
- 1 tablespoon coconut oil or any preferred cooking oil
- 1 large onion, finely chopped
- 3 cloves garlic, minced
- 1 tablespoon grated fresh ginger
- 1 red bell pepper, sliced
- 2 carrots, sliced
- 1 cup cauliflower florets
- 1 cup frozen peas
- 1 can (14 oz) coconut milk
- 2 tablespoons curry powder
- 1 teaspoon ground turmeric
- 1/2 teaspoon ground cumin

- 1/2 teaspoon ground coriander
- 1/4 teaspoon cayenne pepper (adjust to your desired level of spiciness)
- Salt and pepper to taste
- Fresh cilantro leaves for garnish
- Cooked brown rice or quinoa for serving

Instructions:

1. In a large skillet or pot, heat the coconut oil or preferred cooking oil over medium heat.

2. Add the finely chopped onion to the skillet, and sauté until it becomes translucent.

3. Stir in the minced garlic and grated fresh ginger, and sauté for another minute until they release their aromatic fragrance.

4. Add the cubed tofu to the skillet, and cook until it becomes lightly golden on all sides.

5. Stir in the sliced red bell pepper, sliced carrots, cauliflower florets, and frozen peas.

6. In a small bowl, mix the curry powder, ground turmeric, ground cumin, ground coriander, cayenne pepper, salt, and pepper.

7. Sprinkle the curry spice mixture over the vegetables and tofu, stirring everything together to coat the ingredients with the flavorful spices.

8. Pour the coconut milk over the vegetable and tofu mixture, and stir until all the ingredients are well combined.

9. Bring the curry to a gentle simmer, and let it cook for about 15-20 minutes, or until the vegetables are tender and the flavors meld together.

10. Taste the curry and adjust the seasoning, adding more salt, pepper, or curry spices to your liking.

11. Remove the skillet from the heat, and garnish the Tofu and Vegetable Curry with fresh cilantro leaves for a burst of herbal freshness.

12. Serve the aromatic and creamy Tofu and Vegetable Curry over cooked brown rice or quinoa for a wholesome and satisfying meal.

Note: Feel free to customize your curry with other preferred vegetables or adjust the level of spiciness to suit your taste preferences.

Relish the delightful and nutrient-rich Tofu and Vegetable Curry, knowing that you've chosen a dinner that aligns with your A-Negative blood type and provides you with essential nutrients for a satisfying meal. Let's continue our culinary exploration and discover more delightful dinner options to support your overall health and well-being!

Chapter 5:

Satisfying Snacks

- Rice Crackers with Goat Cheese and Cherry Tomatoes

Indulge in a delightful and satisfying snack with our Rice Crackers with Goat Cheese and Cherry Tomatoes—a scrumptious A-Negative-friendly treat that combines the crispiness of rice crackers with the creamy tang of goat cheese and the juicy sweetness of cherry tomatoes. This snack not only tantalizes your taste buds but also provides a quick and nutritious pick-me-up.

Health Tip: The Healthy Components of the Major Ingredients

Let's explore the healthy components of the major ingredients in this Rice Crackers with Goat Cheese and Cherry Tomatoes, showcasing how each element contributes to your well-being:

Rice Crackers: Rice crackers are a gluten-free and light alternative to traditional wheat-based crackers. They offer a satisfying crunch and are easy to digest.

Goat Cheese: Goat cheese is lower in lactose and fat than cow's milk cheese, making it a suitable option for some individuals. It provides calcium, protein, and essential minerals.

Cherry Tomatoes: Cherry tomatoes are rich in vitamins A and C, as well as antioxidants. They support eye health, boost immunity, and add natural sweetness to the snack.

Ingredients:
- Rice crackers (gluten-free if desired)
- Goat cheese, softened
- Cherry tomatoes, halved
- Fresh basil leaves, for garnish
- Freshly ground black pepper, to taste

Instructions:

1. Arrange the rice crackers on a serving platter or a snack plate.

2. Spread a dollop of softened goat cheese on each rice cracker, creating a creamy and tangy base.

3. Top the goat cheese with a halved cherry tomato on each cracker, ensuring a burst of juicy sweetness in every bite.

4. Garnish the Rice Crackers with Goat Cheese and Cherry Tomatoes with fresh basil leaves, adding a touch of herbal aroma and visual appeal.

5. Season the snack with a sprinkle of freshly ground black pepper for a hint of spiciness (optional).

6. Serve the delightful and colorful Rice Crackers with Goat Cheese and Cherry Tomatoes as a satisfying snack option for any time of the day.

Note: You can get creative with additional toppings like a drizzle of balsamic glaze, a sprinkle of chives, or a few pine nuts for added texture.

Enjoy the scrumptious and nutrient-rich Rice Crackers with Goat Cheese and Cherry Tomatoes, knowing that you've chosen a snack that aligns with your A-Negative blood type and provides you with essential nutrients for a quick and delightful treat. Let's continue our culinary exploration and discover more satisfying snack options to support your overall health and well-being!

- Edamame with Sea Salt

Indulge in a delightful and nutritious snack with our Edamame with Sea Salt—a simple yet satisfying A-Negative-friendly treat that showcases the natural flavors of edamame enhanced by the subtle touch of sea salt. This snack not only delights your taste buds but also provides a wholesome boost of protein and essential nutrients.

Health Tip: The Healthy Components of Edamame

Let's explore the healthy components of edamame, showcasing how this delightful snack contributes to your well-being:

Edamame: Edamame, young and green soybeans, are a rich source of plant-based protein, fiber, vitamins, and minerals. They provide essential amino acids, support muscle health, and promote digestion.

Sea Salt: Sea salt is a natural and unprocessed alternative to regular table salt. In moderation, sea salt provides essential minerals like potassium and magnesium and adds flavor to the snack.

Ingredients:
- Edamame in the pod (fresh or frozen)
- Sea salt (coarse or fine), to taste

Instructions:

1. If using frozen edamame, follow the package instructions to cook them until tender. If using fresh edamame, blanch them in boiling water for 2-3 minutes, then drain.

2. Once cooked and tender, transfer the edamame to a serving bowl.

3. Sprinkle sea salt over the edamame, adjusting the amount to your taste preferences. A light dusting of sea salt enhances the natural flavors of the edamame.

4. Toss the edamame gently to ensure the sea salt is evenly distributed.

5. Serve the delightful and protein-rich Edamame with Sea Salt as a wholesome snack option for any time of the day.

Note: You can enjoy edamame as a warm or chilled snack, depending on your preference. If serving chilled, you can rinse the cooked edamame under cold water before sprinkling with sea salt.

Relish the delicious and nutrient-rich Edamame with Sea Salt, knowing that you've chosen a snack that aligns with your A-Negative blood type and provides you with essential nutrients for a quick and delightful treat. Let's continue our culinary exploration and discover more satisfying snack options to support your overall health and well-being!

- Sliced Apples with Almond Butter

Delight in a wholesome and delicious snack with our Sliced Apples with Almond Butter—a delightful A-Negative-friendly treat that combines the natural sweetness of sliced apples with the creamy richness of almond butter. This snack not only satisfies your sweet cravings but also provides a nutritious and energizing pick-me-up.

Health Tip: The Healthy Components of the Snack

Let's explore the healthy components of this Sliced Apples with Almond Butter snack, showcasing how each element contributes to your well-being:

Apples: Apples are a rich source of dietary fiber, vitamins, and antioxidants. They support digestive health, promote heart health, and provide a natural burst of sweetness.

Almond Butter: Almond butter is a nutritious nut butter made from ground almonds. It offers healthy fats, protein, and essential minerals like magnesium and calcium. Almond butter supports brain health, aids in muscle function, and adds creaminess to the snack.

Ingredients:
- Fresh and crisp apples (any preferred variety), sliced
- Natural almond butter (unsweetened and without added oils)

- Optional toppings: A sprinkle of cinnamon, a drizzle of honey (optional for added sweetness), or a few crushed nuts for added crunch

Instructions:

1. Wash and slice the apples into thin and manageable pieces, removing any seeds or cores.

2. Arrange the apple slices on a serving plate or platter.

3. In a small bowl, stir the natural almond butter to ensure it is well mixed.

4. Using a knife or a small spoon, generously spread the almond butter on each apple slice.

5. If desired, add a sprinkle of cinnamon for a warm and comforting flavor.

6. For a touch of sweetness, you can drizzle a little honey over the almond butter (optional).

7. For added crunch and texture, you can sprinkle crushed nuts like almonds or walnuts on top.

8. Serve the wholesome and delectable Sliced Apples with Almond Butter as a satisfying snack option for a quick energy boost.

Note: You can get creative with the toppings by adding a dash of nutmeg, a sprinkle of chia seeds, or a few raisins for added flavor and nutrition.

Enjoy the delicious and nutrient-rich Sliced Apples with Almond Butter, knowing that you've chosen a snack that aligns with your A-Negative blood type and provides you with essential nutrients for a delightful and energizing treat. Let's continue our culinary exploration and discover more satisfying snack options to support your overall health and well-being!

- Seaweed Snacks

Immerse yourself in the savory goodness of Seaweed Snacks—a delightful and nutritious A-Negative-friendly treat that brings the flavors of the ocean to your palate. These crispy and flavorful snacks not only satisfy your cravings but also provide a wealth of essential vitamins and minerals for a guilt-free indulgence.

Health Tip: The Healthy Components of Seaweed Snacks

Let's explore the healthy components of Seaweed Snacks, showcasing how this unique snack contributes to your well-being:

Seaweed (Nori): Seaweed is a nutrient-dense marine plant that is rich in iodine, iron, calcium, and various vitamins. It supports thyroid function, strengthens bones, and promotes overall vitality.

Ingredients:
- Roasted seaweed sheets (nori sheets)

Instructions:

1. Purchase roasted seaweed sheets (nori sheets) from your local grocery store or Asian market. Ensure they are free from added oils and seasonings for a wholesome snack option.

2. Open the package of roasted seaweed sheets, and you'll find thin and delicate seaweed squares.

3. Carefully peel one seaweed sheet from the stack, being gentle to avoid tearing.

4. Place the seaweed sheet on a clean and dry surface, and marvel at its rich green color and oceanic aroma.

5. With your fingers or a clean pair of scissors, cut the seaweed sheet into smaller bite-sized pieces. You can cut them into squares, rectangles, or any preferred shape.

6. Arrange the bite-sized seaweed pieces on a serving plate or a snack bowl.

7. Indulge in the crispy and savory Seaweed Snacks one piece at a time, savoring the unique umami taste and delicate texture.

Note: You can enjoy Seaweed Snacks on their own for a light and refreshing snack or pair them with other A-Negative-friendly treats like sliced cucumbers or radishes for added crunch.

Relish the delightful and nutrient-rich Seaweed Snacks, knowing that you've chosen a snack that aligns with your A-Negative blood type and provides you with essential nutrients for a guilt-free indulgence. Let's continue our culinary exploration and discover more satisfying snack options to support your overall health and well-being!

Chapter 6:

Divine Desserts

- Rice Pudding with Coconut Milk

Satisfy your sweet tooth with a delightful and creamy Rice Pudding with Coconut Milk—a heavenly A-Negative-friendly dessert that combines the comforting flavors of rice and coconut in a velvety, indulgent treat. This dessert not only delights your taste buds but also provides a touch of exotic charm to your culinary experience.

Health Tip: The Healthy Components of the Dessert

Let's explore the healthy components of the Rice Pudding with Coconut Milk, showcasing how this divine dessert contributes to your well-being:

Rice: Rice is a naturally gluten-free grain that offers a source of carbohydrates and energy. It provides a sense of comfort and satisfaction in this dessert.

Coconut Milk: Coconut milk adds a rich and luscious texture to the dessert. It contains medium-chain fatty acids that are easily metabolized for energy, and it's a source of essential minerals like manganese.

Ingredients:
- 1 cup cooked white or brown rice (choose a rice variety that you prefer)
- 1 can (13.5 oz) full-fat coconut milk
- 1/4 cup maple syrup or honey (adjust to your desired level of sweetness)
- 1 teaspoon vanilla extract
- A pinch of salt
- Ground cinnamon, for garnish (optional)
- Toasted coconut flakes, for garnish (optional)

Instructions:
1. In a medium saucepan, combine the cooked rice, full-fat coconut milk, and maple syrup or honey over medium heat.

2. Stir the mixture gently until it comes to a simmer. Lower the heat to medium-low, and continue to cook the rice pudding for about 15-20 minutes, stirring occasionally.

3. As the rice absorbs the coconut milk and thickens, the pudding will develop a creamy and velvety texture.

4. Stir in the vanilla extract and a pinch of salt to enhance the flavors of the dessert.

5. Once the Rice Pudding with Coconut Milk reaches your desired consistency and the rice is tender, remove the saucepan from the heat.

6. Serve the warm and luscious Rice Pudding with Coconut Milk in individual dessert bowls or small cups.

7. If desired, garnish each serving with a sprinkle of ground cinnamon for a warm and aromatic touch.

8. For an extra layer of texture and flavor, top the dessert with toasted coconut flakes, adding a delightful crunch.

9. Enjoy the divine and indulgent Rice Pudding with Coconut Milk as a delightful dessert to satisfy your sweet cravings.

Note: You can adjust the sweetness of the dessert by adding more or less maple syrup or honey according to your taste preferences.

Savor the delightful and creamy Rice Pudding with Coconut Milk, knowing that you've chosen a dessert that aligns with your A-Negative blood type and provides you with a touch of exotic charm in every spoonful. Let's continue our culinary exploration and discover more divine dessert options to support your overall health and well-being!

- Baked Apples with Cinnamon and Honey

Indulge in the warm and comforting flavors of Baked Apples with Cinnamon and Honey—a delightful A-Negative-friendly dessert that elevates the natural sweetness of apples with a touch of aromatic cinnamon and a drizzle of golden honey. This dessert not only warms your heart but also provides a wholesome and guilt-free treat.

Health Tip: The Healthy Components of the Dessert

Let's explore the healthy components of Baked Apples with Cinnamon and Honey, showcasing how this divine dessert contributes to your well-being:

Apples: Apples are a rich source of dietary fiber, vitamins, and antioxidants. They support digestive health, promote heart health, and provide a natural burst of sweetness.

Cinnamon: Cinnamon adds a warm and comforting aroma to the dessert. It contains antioxidants and has been linked to potential health benefits, including improved blood sugar regulation.

Honey: Honey offers natural sweetness and a touch of decadence to the dessert. Opt for raw and unprocessed honey to enjoy its potential health benefits.

Ingredients:
- Apples (any preferred variety), cored and halved
- Ground cinnamon
- Raw and unprocessed honey

Instructions:

1. Preheat your oven to 375°F (190°C).

2. Wash the apples thoroughly, and remove the cores using an apple corer or a small knife. Halve the apples to create a flat surface for baking.

3. Place the halved apples on a baking sheet or in a baking dish, cut-side up.

4. Generously sprinkle ground cinnamon over each apple half, coating them in the warm and aromatic spice.

5. Drizzle a small amount of raw and unprocessed honey over the cinnamon-coated apples. The honey adds a delightful sweetness to the dessert.

6. Place the baking sheet or dish in the preheated oven, and bake the apples for approximately 20-25 minutes or until they become tender.

7. As the apples bake, the cinnamon and honey will infuse the fruit with delightful flavors.

8. Once the Baked Apples with Cinnamon and Honey are done baking, remove them from the oven.

9. Serve the warm and fragrant Baked Apples with Cinnamon and Honey as a comforting dessert option for a cozy and satisfying treat.

Note: You can enjoy the Baked Apples with Cinnamon and Honey on their own or pair them with a dollop of Greek yogurt or a scoop of vanilla ice cream for added indulgence.

Relish the delightful and wholesome Baked Apples with Cinnamon and Honey, knowing that you've chosen a dessert that aligns with your A-Negative blood type and provides you with a comforting and delicious treat. Let's continue our culinary exploration and discover more divine dessert options to support your overall health and well-being!

- Mixed Berry Sorbet

Delight in the refreshing and vibrant flavors of Mixed Berry Sorbet—a delightful A-Negative-friendly dessert that celebrates the natural sweetness of a medley of berries in a cool and velvety treat. This sorbet not only pleases your palate but also provides a burst of antioxidants and essential vitamins for a guilt-free indulgence.

Health Tip: The Healthy Components of the Dessert

Let's explore the healthy components of Mixed Berry Sorbet, showcasing how this divine dessert contributes to your well-being:

Mixed Berries: Berries like strawberries, blueberries, raspberries, and blackberries are rich in antioxidants, vitamins, and dietary fiber. They promote heart health, boost immunity, and support healthy skin.

Ingredients:
- 2 cups mixed berries (fresh or frozen), such as strawberries, blueberries, raspberries, and blackberries
- 1/4 cup natural sweetener (maple syrup, honey, or agave syrup) (adjust according to your taste preferences)
- 1 tablespoon freshly squeezed lemon juice

- Fresh mint leaves, for garnish (optional)

Instructions:

1. If using frozen mixed berries, let them thaw slightly at room temperature for a few minutes.

2. In a blender or food processor, add the mixed berries, natural sweetener of your choice, and freshly squeezed lemon juice.

3. Blend the mixture until smooth and well combined, creating a luscious and vibrant berry puree.

4. Taste the berry puree and adjust the sweetness by adding more natural sweetener if desired.

5. Once the berry puree is smooth and sweetened to your liking, transfer it to a shallow container or a loaf pan.

6. Cover the container with a lid or plastic wrap, and place it in the freezer for about 4-6 hours or until the sorbet becomes firm.

7. Every 30 minutes during the freezing process, take the sorbet out of the freezer and give it a gentle stir with a fork. This step ensures a smooth and creamy texture.

8. Once the Mixed Berry Sorbet is fully frozen and set, remove it from the freezer.

9. Use an ice cream scoop or a spoon to serve the sorbet in individual dessert bowls or glasses.

10. For an elegant touch, garnish each serving with fresh mint leaves, adding a burst of herbal freshness.

11. Enjoy the refreshing and nutrient-rich Mixed Berry Sorbet as a delightful dessert option to cool down and rejuvenate on warm days.

Note: You can customize this sorbet with other preferred berries or add a dash of vanilla extract for a hint of aromatic flavor.

Savor the delightful and rejuvenating Mixed Berry Sorbet, knowing that you've chosen a dessert that aligns with your A-Negative blood type and provides you with a refreshing and nourishing treat. Let's continue our culinary exploration and discover more divine dessert options to support your overall health and well-being!

- Carob Chip Cookies with Oat Flour

Indulge in the delectable and wholesome goodness of Carob Chip Cookies with Oat Flour—a delightful A-Negative-friendly dessert that combines the rich flavors of carob chips with the heartiness of oat flour for a chewy and satisfying treat. These cookies not only satisfy your sweet cravings but also provide a healthier twist to a classic favorite.

Health Tip: The Healthy Components of the Cookies

Let's explore the healthy components of Carob Chip Cookies with Oat Flour, showcasing how these divine cookies contribute to your well-being:

Oat Flour: Oat flour is a nutritious alternative to traditional all-purpose flour. It offers dietary fiber, protein, and essential minerals like manganese and phosphorus.

Carob Chips: Carob chips are a naturally sweet and caffeine-free alternative to chocolate chips. They are a source of antioxidants, calcium, and fiber.

Ingredients:
- 1 cup oat flour (you can blend rolled oats into a fine powder to make oat flour)
- 1/2 teaspoon baking soda
- A pinch of salt
- 1/4 cup coconut oil or butter, melted

- 1/4 cup natural sweetener (maple syrup, honey, or coconut sugar) (adjust according to your taste preferences)
- 1 teaspoon vanilla extract
- 1/4 cup carob chips (ensure they are free from added sugars)
- 1/4 cup chopped nuts (walnuts or almonds) (optional for added crunch)

Instructions:

1. Preheat your oven to 350°F (175°C), and line a baking sheet with parchment paper.

2. In a mixing bowl, whisk together the oat flour, baking soda, and a pinch of salt.

3. In a separate microwave-safe bowl or on the stovetop, melt the coconut oil or butter.

4. Stir the natural sweetener and vanilla extract into the melted coconut oil or butter, creating a smooth and liquid mixture.

5. Pour the wet ingredients into the bowl of dry ingredients, and mix until they are well combined.

6. Fold in the carob chips, ensuring they are evenly distributed throughout the cookie dough.

7. If desired, add chopped nuts to the cookie dough for an extra layer of crunch and texture.

8. Using a spoon or your hands, portion the cookie dough into small balls and place them on the lined baking sheet.

9. Gently press down each cookie dough ball to create a cookie shape, keeping some space between each cookie.

10. Bake the Carob Chip Cookies with Oat Flour in the preheated oven for approximately 10-12 minutes or until the edges turn golden brown.

11. Once the cookies are baked to perfection, remove the baking sheet from the oven.

12. Allow the cookies to cool on the baking sheet for a few minutes before transferring them to a wire rack to cool completely.

13. Serve the delicious and chewy Carob Chip Cookies with Oat Flour as a delightful dessert or snack option for a guilt-free indulgence.

Note: You can customize these cookies with other additions like dried fruits, shredded coconut, or a sprinkle of cinnamon for added flavor.

Relish the delectable and nutrient-rich Carob Chip Cookies with Oat Flour, knowing that you've chosen a dessert that aligns with your A-Negative blood type and provides you with a wholesome and satisfying treat. Let's continue our culinary exploration and discover more divine dessert options to support your overall health and well-being!

Chapter 7

- Tips for Successful Meal Planning and Preparation

Meal planning and preparation are essential for maintaining a healthy and balanced diet that aligns with your A-Negative blood type. By thoughtfully organizing your meals, you can make nutritious choices and avoid impromptu unhealthy options. Here are some valuable tips to help you succeed in your meal planning and preparation journey:

1. Know Your Blood Type Diet:
Familiarize yourself with the principles of the Blood Type Diet for A-Negative. Understand the foods that are beneficial and those to avoid, allowing you to create meals that support your specific nutritional needs.

2. Create a Weekly Menu:
Design a weekly meal plan that includes a variety of A-Negative-friendly dishes.

Incorporate whole grains, lean proteins, fruits, vegetables, and healthy fats into your menu to ensure a well-rounded diet.

3. Utilize Seasonal Ingredients:
Make the most of seasonal produce when planning your meals. Seasonal fruits and vegetables are often more flavorful and cost-effective.

4. Pre-Cook and Store:
Consider pre-cooking certain components of your meals, such as grains, proteins, and sauces. Store them in separate containers in the refrigerator or freezer for easy assembly during the week.

5. Batch Cooking:
Prepare larger quantities of certain dishes, like soups, stews, or casseroles, to enjoy throughout the week. Batch cooking saves time and ensures you always have a healthy meal option on hand.

6. Smart Grocery Shopping:
Compile a shopping list based on your weekly menu and stick to it when grocery shopping.

Avoid impulse purchases of unhealthy snacks or foods that don't align with your blood type diet.

7. Portion Control:
Practice portion control to avoid overeating and to manage your calorie intake. Remember that a balanced diet is about quality and quantity.

8. Invest in Quality Containers:
Invest in good-quality food storage containers to keep your prepped ingredients and leftovers fresh for an extended period.

9. Embrace Food Safety:
Practice proper food safety protocols to prevent foodborne illnesses. Wash your hands, clean cooking surfaces, and store perishables at appropriate temperatures.

10. Experiment with New Recipes:
Don't be afraid to try new A-Negative-friendly recipes to keep your meals exciting and enjoyable. Look for creative ways to incorporate flavors and textures that align with your blood type diet.

11. Listen to Your Body:

Pay attention to how your body responds to different foods. Everyone's dietary needs may vary, so listen to your body and adjust your meal planning accordingly.

12. Stay Hydrated:

Remember to drink plenty of water throughout the day. Hydration is essential for overall well-being and supports your body's functions.

By implementing these tips, you can make meal planning and preparation a seamless and enjoyable part of your lifestyle. Embrace the benefits of the Blood Type Diet for A-Negative and nourish your body with wholesome and delicious meals tailored to your specific needs. Happy and healthy eating!

- Embracing a Healthy Lifestyle with the Blood Type A Diet

The Blood Type A Diet offers a personalized approach to nutrition, tailored specifically to individuals with A-Negative blood type. Embracing this healthy lifestyle goes beyond meal planning and preparation—it involves making mindful choices that support your overall well-being. Here are essential tips to help you fully embrace a healthy lifestyle with the Blood Type A Diet:

1. Understand Your Blood Type:

Educate yourself about the characteristics and unique nutritional requirements of A-Negative blood type. Knowing the science behind the diet will empower you to make informed decisions about your food choices.

2. Prioritize Plant-Based Foods:

Focus on incorporating a wide variety of nutrient-dense, plant-based foods into your meals. Fresh fruits, vegetables, legumes, and whole grains should form the foundation of your diet.

3. Choose Lean Proteins:
Opt for lean protein sources like tofu, tempeh, lentils, and beans. These plant-based proteins are well-suited to your blood type and provide essential nutrients.

4. Avoid Processed Foods:
Minimize or eliminate processed and refined foods from your diet. These items are often high in added sugars, unhealthy fats, and artificial ingredients that may not align with the Blood Type A Diet.

5. Practice Mindful Eating:
Eat slowly and savor each bite to fully enjoy your meals. Mindful eating can help prevent overeating and improve digestion.

6. Incorporate Gentle Exercise:
Engage in low-impact exercises like yoga, Pilates, walking, or swimming to promote physical health and reduce stress.

7. Manage Stress:

Stress can impact your overall well-being and digestion. Incorporate stress-relief practices into your routine, such as meditation, deep breathing exercises, or spending time in nature.

8. Stay Hydrated:

Ensure you drink an adequate amount of water throughout the day to support your body's functions and maintain hydration.

9. Get Quality Sleep:

Aim for 7-9 hours of quality sleep each night to support your body's recovery and overall health.

10. Regular Health Checkups:

Visit your healthcare provider regularly for checkups and to monitor your health. Discuss your dietary choices and any concerns you may have.

11. Enjoy Balanced Treats:

While following the Blood Type A Diet, it's okay to indulge in balanced treats occasionally. Look for healthier dessert options that align with your blood type.

12. Build a Support System:
Surround yourself with supportive friends or family who understand and respect your dietary choices. Having a strong support system can make the journey more enjoyable.

By embracing a healthy lifestyle that aligns with the Blood Type A Diet, you are making a conscious effort to prioritize your health and well-being. As you cultivate these habits, you'll notice positive changes in your energy levels, digestion, and overall vitality. Remember that every step toward a healthier lifestyle is a step toward a more vibrant and fulfilling life. Keep learning, experimenting, and enjoying the journey to optimal health!

Conclusion

Congratulations on completing your journey through the Blood Type A Cookbook! You've embarked on a delightful culinary adventure tailored specifically to A-Positive and A-Negative blood types, discovering a world of delicious and nutritious recipes that support your well-being. This cookbook was designed to provide you with a friendly and informative guide to create wholesome meals that align with your unique nutritional needs.

Throughout this cookbook, you've explored a diverse array of breakfast delights, scrumptious lunches, delectable dinners, satisfying snacks, and divine desserts—all thoughtfully curated to complement your A-Positive or A-Negative blood type. Each recipe came with human-like explanations, highlighting the health benefits of ingredients and how they contribute to your overall health.

But beyond the recipes, you've also delved into the basics of the Blood Type Diet, understanding what makes your blood type unique and how it influences your dietary choices. By embracing the Blood Type A Diet, you've taken a step toward nourishing your body in a way that supports optimal health and well-being.

Remember, the journey to a healthier lifestyle doesn't end with this cookbook. Continue to explore new recipes, experiment with flavors, and embrace the principles of the Blood Type Diet. As you prioritize plant-based foods, lean proteins, and mindful eating, you'll notice positive changes in your energy levels, digestion, and overall vitality.

We hope this cookbook has ignited your passion for healthful cooking and empowered you to make informed choices about the foods you consume. Whether you're preparing meals for yourself, your family, or friends, the Blood Type A Cookbook has equipped you with the knowledge and inspiration to create nourishing and delicious dishes.

As you continue on your journey to better health, remember to listen to your body, stay curious, and cultivate a supportive community that values your commitment to a healthy lifestyle. Embrace the joy of cooking and relish in the satisfaction of knowing you're nurturing your body in the best way possible.

Thank you for joining us on this culinary adventure, and may you enjoy a lifetime of health, happiness, and delicious meals tailored to your unique blood type.

Happy cooking and bon appétit!

Printed in Great Britain
by Amazon

41401080R00136